YOUR PAIN IS
REAL

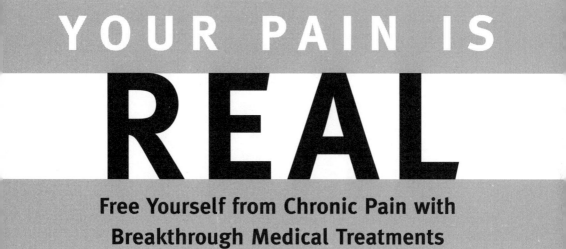

YOUR PAIN IS
REAL

Free Yourself from Chronic Pain with Breakthrough Medical Treatments

DR. EMILE HIESIGER

with Kathleen Brady

ReganBooks

An Imprint of HarperCollins*Publishers*

This book is meant to educate readers about the causes of pain and guide them in seeking appropriate care. It is not meant to replace medical consultation and treatment. The author and the publisher disclaim responsibility for any adverse effects arising from the use or application of the information contained in this book. The use of particular brand names is not to be construed as an advertisement for or endorsement of one commercially available product over another. Examples of commercial brand names have been used for the convenience of the reader, as they are easier to pronounce than generic names. The names of patients, whose stories are accurately recounted, have been changed to preserve their privacy.

FIRST EDITION

Printed on acid-free paper

Designed by Jessica Shatan
Illustrations by the author

Library of Congress Cataloging-in-Publication Data
Hiesiger, Emile.
    Your pain is real : free yourself from chronic pain with breakthrough medical treatments / Emile Hiesiger, with Kathleen Brady.
        p.   cm.
    Includes index.
    ISBN 0-06-039324-6
    1. Chronic pain—Popular works.   I. Brady, Kathleen.   II. Title.
RB127 .H54 2001
616'.0472—dc21   00-047017

01 02 03 04 05   RRD   10 9 8 7 6 5 4 3 2 1

I dedicate this book to my patients, who have taught me more about pain than any textbook, lecture, or professor.

I dedicate the chapter on spinal disorders to Dr. Vallo Benjamin, an outstanding neurosurgeon and devoted friend, who patiently and kindly taught me about various surgical disorders affecting the spine, the use and interpretation of radiological studies to diagnose them, and their treatment through conservative surgery. He also impressed upon me the importance of outcome analysis in determining the success or failure of everything we do in medicine—but especially following any intervention where the physician may not have long-term contact with the patient. This includes the period, however long, following surgery and pain-relieving procedures. I also thank him for his considerable help in the growth of my career.

CONTENTS

Acknowledgments xi

Foreword xiii

Introduction xv

1 UNCOVERING THE MYSTERIES OF CHRONIC PHYSICAL PAIN

The Chronic Undertreatment of Chronic Pain   3
Pathways of Pain: How Your Body Gets the Message   4
How Your Body Modulates Pain Naturally   5
How We Think About and Feel Pain   9
Variations in the Way We Perceive Pain   10
When the System Runs Amok: Sensitization   11
Referred Pain: Why the Cause Is Not Always Near the Effect   13
Test-Negative Pain: When the Cause Can't Be Seen   14
Key Points in Getting Your Pain Correctly Diagnosed   16

2 CONTROLLING PAIN WITHOUT MEDICATION OR SURGERY

Lifestyle Changes   18
Nonmedical Pain Management   25
Alternative and Complementary Medicine   33
Key Points About Nonmedical Pain Management   38

3 MEDICATION IN THE TREATMENT OF PAIN

The Challenge of Finding the Drug That Works   41
Treating Pain with Narcotics   50

Methods of Delivery   58
Medication and Aging   61
Key Points About Medication for Pain   63

4   HEADACHES FROM HELL AND OTHER PAINS
ABOVE THE NECK

Migraines: Stop Pounding on My Head   65
Cluster Headaches: Get That Ice Pick out of My Eye!   69
Tension Headaches: Please Loosen the Headband!   71
Rebound Headaches: The Cure Is Killing Me   71
Post-traumatic Headaches   72
When to See a Headache Specialist   73
Atypical Facial Pain   75
Jaws: Temporomandibular Joint Syndrome (TMJ)   76
Head Trauma   78
Key Points About Head Pain   84

5   TREATING PAINFUL MUSCLES, BONES, AND JOINTS

Myofascial Pain   85
Spasms and Cramps   88
When Painful Muscles Signal a Deeper Problem   89
The Enigma of Fibromyalgia   90
Osteoarthritis: Wear and Tear on the Joints   92
Rheumatoid Arthritis: The Body at War with Itself   94
Osteoporosis: The Pain of Disintegrating Bones   95
Key Points About Musculoskeletal Pain   100

6   YOUR ACHING BACK: PAIN FROM HEAD TO TOE

How Wear and Tear Creates Pain   104
Low-Back Pain   109
The Diagnostic Challenge of Back Pain   114
Evaluating Your Treatment Options   115
Treating Back Pain with Surgery   124
Key Points About Back Pain   128

7 THE NERVE OF THAT PAIN: NEUROPATHIC PAIN

Painful Twitch: Trigeminal Neuralgia   131
A Tangled Mass of Nerves: Neuromas   135
Diabetic Neuropathy   137
The Neuropathic Pain Syndromes of AIDS/HIV   139
Complex Regional Pain Syndrome (CRPS):
   The Black Hole of Neuropathic Pain   141
Pain Following Shingles: Postherpetic Neuralgia   146
The Spider's Painful Web: Arachnoiditis   149
Pain from Damaged Nerve Roots   150
Stroke or Spinal-Cord-Injury Pain   151
Phantom-Limb Pain   152
Key Points About Neuropathic Pain   157

8 PREVENTION AND TREATMENT OF PAINFUL SPORTS INJURIES

Sprains and Strains   159
Overuse Injuries   161
Stress Fractures   163
Anterior Cruciate Ligament (ACL) Injuries   164
Spinal Injuries   166
Injuries to Nerves   167
Headaches   169
Basic Prevention and Treatment   170
Key Points About Painful Sports Injuries   172

9 GYNECOLOGIC PAIN

Recurrent Pelvic Pain   175
Chronic Pelvic Pain   176
Key Points About Gynecologic Pain   183

10 REDUCING THE PAIN OF CANCER

Pain Following Surgery   187
Radiation Therapy   189

Chemotherapy   191
Treatment with Corticosteroids   192
Treatment with Narcotics and Other Drugs   193
How Cancer Affects the Body's Response
    to Pain Medication   198
Lesioning Nerves to Relieve Pain   198
The Cancer and Pain-Management Team   201
Key Points About Cancer Pain   203

11 HOW TO GET AND PAY FOR THE BEST
TREATMENT FOR PAIN

Getting the Most from Your Health-Insurance Plan   209
Finding the Best Doctor   210
Key Points About Finding the Best Care   218

Afterword   219

Glossary   223

Resources   231

Suggested Reading   239

Index   241

ACKNOWLEDGMENTS

I thank Mrs. Marie Merzon, a patient of mine who kindly performed a critical and helpful reading of the manuscript and who has become a dear friend. She taught me more about referred spinal pain than anyone else I have met in my clinical career. She also is an extraordinary human being who has dogged determination to leave no stone unturned in seeking the treatment that will best allow her to pursue her greatest joy—the challenge of life.

I thank Mr. Ernie Jaffee and Professor Charles Winick for convincing me that I had a book to write. I thank Drs. Ernest Mathews, Lloyd Saberski, and Abraham Chachoua for critically reviewing parts of the manuscript. I thank Professor Emeritus William Breger for his help in critically evaluating the entire manuscript, planning the illustrations, and teaching me tolerance toward the human weaknesses underlying the health-care system in which we live and practice. Professor Breger, architect and health planner, is a wonderful, loving, avuncular friend of many years, who never ceases to inspire me as a role model with his indefatigable love for both the power of logical thought and the creative process.

Several colleagues taught me, early in my career, how to analyze a scientific problem and write scientific material. In this regard, I thank my former collaborators from the PET project at Brookhaven National Laboratory. They are Dr. Jonathan Brodie of New York University; the late Dr. Alfred Wolf, former chairman of the Department of Chemistry, Brookhaven National Laboratory; and Dr. Joanna Fowler of Brookhaven National Laboratory. I also thank Dr. William Shapiro, my mentor while I was at Memorial Sloan-Kettering Cancer Center.

I thank Dr. Albert Goodgold for his friendship, wise and patient counsel, confidence, and help in the growth of my career. I owe great thanks to Dr. Norman Chase, former chairman of the Department of Radiology (retired), and Dr. Phillip Evanski, former acting chairman of the Department of Orthopedics (retired), for allowing me to start performing various radiologically guided procedures at New York University. My thanks also to Dr. Leslie St. Louis and Dr. Alex Bernstein for permitting me to expand my procedural repertoire while working at radiological facilities owned or controlled by them.

I wish to thank my editor at Regan Books, Mr. Douglas Corcoran, for his never-ending constructive criticism, support, and patience with a novice author.

I thank my beloved wife, Patricia, for her unflagging maturity, understanding, encouragement, and patience during the year it took to write this book. During this time she attended, almost single-handedly, to the plans for our lovely wedding, which took place on May 18, 2000, during the final months of work on the book. I also thank Ms. Judy Vargas, my personal secretary, Melinda Tanner, and Maria Santana, the members of my office staff, and my close colleagues for their understanding during the long and often tense period when I was writing the book while conducting a busy practice.

FOREWORD

Chronic pain interferes with the lives of more than thirty-five million American adults. It is responsible for almost as much health-care consumption as the common cold and it costs far more, for medical treatments and in terms of lost wages and human suffering. Patients expect that the doctor will cure them, but this often does not happen.

Americans are the best consumers in the world; we need to turn our consumerism skills to obtaining health care if we are going to relieve the chronic pain epidemic. Dr. Hiesiger has written this book to bring to public attention valuable information about the causes of chronic pain and the opportunities that exist for treatment.

Just as pain is common, so are its treatments. The first step to successful treatment is accurate diagnosis, as Dr. Hiesiger clearly writes. Next, the patient and the health-care provider must select a treatment that has a reasonable likelihood of success and a low incidence of side effects. This book provides information that a consumer will need in making this selection. It discusses a wide array of diseases and treatments. It explains modern concepts of pain and its management so that the reader can visit his or her health-care provider armed with information. Finally, it offers practical tips on how to seek out good health care for chronic pain.

This is not just another self-help book. It is a source of information about chronic pain and about ways to work with health-care professionals as an educated partner, and it is also a guide to obtaining good health care for sufferers of chronic pain. Chronic pain is rarely a problem that can be solved by simple remedies. It takes teamwork among the patient and all of the providers. This book can be an effective part of that process.

—JOHN D. LOESER, M.D.

INTRODUCTION

All interest in disease and death
Is only another expression of interest in life.

—THOMAS MANN, *The Magic Mountain*

Most of the thirty-five million American adults in chronic pain have lived with their pain for an average of five years and a third of them describe that pain as the worst imaginable. Just over half the chronic pain sufferers say their pain is under control. This means there are approximately seventeen million people in uncontrollable pain—every day and every night of their lives. This has a profound effect, physically and emotionally, on the quality of life, not only for the person in pain but for his or her family.

I have been treating pain for more than twenty years. Most of my patients come to me after they have been in pain for many years and, in the pursuit of relief, have tried many doctors and remedies. You will read many of their stories in this book. In fact, the stories are my way of showing you how much attention must be paid and how much work must be done in order to find the particular treatment that is effective for a particular individual.

Writing this book is my attempt to help you find out how your body and mind react to pain, why it is so difficult to diagnose, and why you must never give up. Don't listen to anyone who tells you to "learn to live with it." Pain can be minimized, even when the cause of the pain cannot be removed. Medical science may not be able to cure cancer yet, but we can give strong drugs to ease its pain. We cannot cure advanced osteoporosis, but we can mend cracked bones that cause the pain. We cannot regenerate a damaged nerve, but we can block the pain message it sends to the brain.

Few patients take advantage of the medication, surgery, or less invasive techniques that can help them. Partly this is because so many different kinds of doctors undertreat pain. If you ask me, a neurologist, about drugs to help your heart, I'll tell you about ten. A cardiologist could tell you more than twenty. It is the same in pain management. Doctors who specialize in pain know more about alleviating pain than the doctors who specialize in the diseases that cause pain.

My colleagues and I who try to alleviate pain often have to teach patients and their families that taking medicine is not a sin or a sign of weakness. I have had to coax some particularly stoic but severely suffering patients to try not to be unduly brave or considerate to those around them by not complaining. I want you to complain. Tell your family members and me when you are in pain. I need to know whether a treatment is working or has stopped working, or never worked at all, and I will only know that if you tell me.

Pain, especially chronic pain, is a subjective phenomenon, tied up in historical Judeo-Christian concepts such as the nobility of quiet suffering, the need for bodily punishment to expiate sins (think of the hair shirt!), and psychosomatic medicine. Pain is colored by skepticism and moral judgment, and it is often second-guessed by armchair psychologists.

If you are in pain, you need to take medicine and use treatments that help you effectively and efficiently. Taking medications to ease pain is no different than taking medication for asthma or high blood pressure. Unfortunately, for a host of cultural reasons, pain and its treatment, especially with narcotics, are viewed differently than medical complaints, the causes of which are easy for a doctor to find with tests.

Pain anywhere in the body should be treated early and aggressively with whatever works. Depending on the type of pain, treatment may start with simple remedies like Tylenol (acetaminophen), ice packs, exercise, physical therapy, or even something like a course of acupuncture, if you choose to try alternative or complementary medicines. If the pain persists, see a pain specialist and find out what is wrong. Depending on the diagnosis—and a correct one may take some time—you have options from drugs through a range of other therapies outlined in this book.

A sensible person would not use a bulldozer to hammer a nail, nor would he or she reach for morphine at the first sign of a headache. Your doctor won't, either. In pain management, we progress from the simplest, easiest means of getting relief on up to more complicated ones. The process is not unlike climbing a ladder.

There are many stories in this book about climbing that ladder, about the trial and error of finding the best treatment for the unique individual. There are stories of impossible pain and seemingly impossible cures for that pain.

The alleviation or cure of pain, particularly when it is of long duration, is an art as well as a science. There is no magic bullet, but there is an arsenal of weapons, small and large, that can fight a successful war against chronic pain—a war that you may have to wage all your life.

To me, medicine is still a special and noble profession. My entire professional obligation is to my patients—never to an insurance company, particular hospital, other physician, or medical school. This old-fashioned philosophy has not made me politically popular in some circles, but it has allowed me hopefully to gain the respect of my patients and like-minded colleagues, and has allowed me to go to sleep with peace of mind every night.

If I have been successful with this book, it should help you understand that you don't have to live in pain, but that you must seek out excellent medical care—and pay for it. (You can fight the insurance companies, by the way.) You must stay connected to the people you love and the work that gratifies you.

Here's to life, a life without pain.

YOUR PAIN IS
REAL

1

Uncovering the Mysteries of Chronic Physical Pain

Pain has an element of blank;
It cannot recollect
When it began, or if there were
A day when it was not.

It has no future but itself,
Its infinite realms contain
Its past, enlightened to perceive
New periods of pain.

—EMILY DICKINSON, "The Mystery of Pain"

My patients have very precise ways of describing their pain to me. "It feels like there's a hot iron in my foot," one says. Some perceive their pain in horrifying, vivid terms, like being ripped up by a pack of guard dogs. To others, their pain may feel like deliberately inflicted torture, like the slow *drip, drip* of water on the forehead until it seems like a sledgehammer. When someone tells me, "It feels like I've been kicked by a horse," I know he is in pain, whether or not actual bodily damage is occurring. Our descriptive ability has a very real foundation in the mysterious way our body and brain monitor pain—but we'll get to that in a minute.

Pain may be the predominant symptom of a condition like a tension headache or a manifestation of a disease like cancer or rheumatoid arthritis. However, the subjective nature of pain makes it a challenge to understand and treat. The inability to verify the presence of pain or measure objectively its severity leads to an insufficient understanding and treatment of pain complaints by society, including family, friends, the medical profession, and insurance companies.

There are various types of pain, and each type is usually described differently.

- *Musculoskeletal pain* is the most common. It is the aching often associated with arthritis, fibromyalgia, most back and neck pain, some headaches, temporomandibular joint (jaw) dysfunction, and cancer pain.

- *Visceral pain* is colicky, often associated with intestinal or stomach problems and with some abdominal cancers.

- *Neuropathic pain* is burning, shocklike, tingling, and at times aching, and is caused by damage to or dysfunction of nerves, such as stroke, neuralgias, neuropathies, sciatica, failed spinal surgery, toothaches, and some cancers.

Pain may be short-lived (acute), of intermediate duration (sub-acute), long-lived (chronic), or chronic with acute flare-ups. Acute pain is localized, lasts from hours to days, and is most common during and after childbirth and following surgery or trauma like breaking a leg. Acute pain usually has a clearly identifiable cause and is associated with wincing, screaming, increased sweating, and elevated blood pressure.

Sub-acute pain is intermediate in duration, lasting a few weeks, like recovery from a hysterectomy. Acute and sub-acute pain are usually treated effectively with nonsteroidal medication like aspirin and, when severe, narcotics. However, even though most physicians can now treat acute pain effectively, there are still some who undertreat—especially with drugs—this most observable and treatable of pain.

Chronic pain tends to be more diffuse than acute pain and often extends well beyond the original painful site. For example, pain from the burn of a match initially is localized to the actual burn site. Then the area around the burn becomes red, swollen, and sensitive. Similarly, in chronic pain, a damaged or scarred nerve (neuroma) initially causes localized pain, but over time, the area surrounding the damage becomes supersensitive, even to the lightest touch, which may be perceived as electric-shock-like pain. Following a car accident, body areas outside the area of the initial local trauma may become chronically painful.

Acute pain has a definite survival value. It tells us to get away from a particular painful stimulus, whatever hurt us. If we live to confront that stimulus again, pain acts as a potent aid in learning "not to do that again." Getting a finger burned by a hot coal on a fire is how children learn about the painful aspect of the alluring glow of the red-orange coals and the bright crackling orange and yellow flames. Chronic pain, on the other hand, has no apparent survival value. It exists independent of a readily observable stimulus. It often means "the system is broken." In primitive society, and perhaps even in developing countries, it is a detriment to survival. In developed countries it represents a black cloud that follows its victim, impairing his or her success and well-being.

Chronic pain is more challenging to treat than acute pain for many reasons. For one, we cannot always find the source of the pain easily, and if we cannot treat it with lifestyle changes or medications, then more invasive therapies have to be tried. For example, with nerve-blocking procedures; nervous system stimulators that mask pain behind a buzzing feeling; implanted pumps delivering medication directly into the fluid around the spinal cord and brain; or the destruction of nerves carrying pain messages. Surgery may be necessary when it is the best way we can remove the cause of the pain, such as a spinal disk pressing on a nerve.

The focus of this book is that elusive and mysterious pain that keeps more than thirty-five million Americans in physical and often emotional agony. It can be hard to find the source of the pain, and so it tends to be blamed on psychological causes when doctors can't find a physiological cause. Physical pain, especially of long duration, frequently results in psychological pain—anxiety and depression. People's lives can be ruined because they enter—or are forced into—a downward spiral of incorrect diagnoses, untreated pain, disability, depression, more pain and suffering, and on and on.

THE CHRONIC UNDERTREATMENT OF CHRONIC PAIN

Chronic pain is often grossly undertreated by the medical profession, which better understands pain that has a clear basis. Doctors like to see an abnormal MRI revealing a tumor invading bone or an electrical nerve study showing a severe neuropathy (Eureka!) rather than hear a patient describe pain with no verifiable information.

People whose severe pain has a basis that cannot be seen or measured (see "Test-Negative Pain" on page 14) are in many cases dismissed as fakes or accused of having a psychological problem. There are a host of painful conditions for which there are no better initial diagnostic tools than a patient's history and a good physical examination. Headaches

is types of spine pain, for example, are like this. So is pain
trauma like whiplash. These test-negative conditions are
treatable through medication, physical therapy, and pain-
relieving procedures, but physicians not directly involved in the treatment of pain often cannot recognize or treat these conditions.

Chronic pain syndrome affects every aspect of life. It may lead to
depression, anxiety, social and financial problems, and even spiritual
difficulties. When you are being evaluated for any pain problem, both
you and your physician owe it to each other to assess both the physical and psychological components of the symptoms and treat both. Becoming permanently disabled must be avoided at all costs. Once you
descend down the smooth glassy funnel into the inferno of disability,
it is almost impossible to climb out. Then, faced with the loss not only
of your livelihood but of your sense of well-being, you can also lose
the ability to correct whatever causes the pain and treat it effectively.

PATHWAYS OF PAIN: HOW YOUR BODY GETS THE MESSAGE

The nervous system is a series of fascinating feedback loops. Once a
pain is detected anywhere in the body, an electrical impulse is fired off
to the brain to let it know what's happening. The brain mobilizes immediately to send other impulses back down to the body to try to
moderate the pain. It was because of my love for this marvelous and
complex "master system" that I decided to study clinical neuroscience.
I wanted to be able to manipulate this incredibly intricate system to
overcome suffering from either the proper *function* or *malfunction* of
the nervous system. Pain arises for either of these two reasons. Let's
see if I can give you the gist of how the system works so you'll have a
better understanding of how and why you are in pain.

Think of the nervous system as an upside-down tree. The roots and
trunk represent the central nervous system—the brain and spinal cord,
respectively. The trunk of the tree (spinal cord) is composed of bundles of nerves that relay information between the roots (brain) and
branches and leaves (peripheral nervous system), which goes out to the
rest of the body. At the end of the branches are the leaves—the peripheral nerve endings that detect sensory information, which are
called receptors. The receptors are located throughout the body: skin,
muscles, blood vessels, joints, eyes, ears, bladder—all the organs. Receptors receive the first information about sensations, including pain,
but they don't actually feel pain. They register the intensity of pressure

(having your foot stepped on), heat or cold, and chemical irritation (cleaning a cut with alcohol), and they create electrical impulses in proportion to the sensation received. More pain means firing off more impulses. Think of the difference between a human and a large horse stepping on your foot.

Pain impulses are transmitted from the body to the spinal cord by one long nerve cell, from the spinal cord to the brain by another long nerve cell, and subsequently to various parts of the brain by multiple short nerve cells. The nerve cells are called neurons. The brain is the processing center, governing your perception of and reaction to pain. Deep in the center of the brain, the thalamus is an enormous relay center, like an airline hub, but far more complex and efficient than O'Hare Airport. It sends all sorts of incoming information about pain to other parts of the brain for processing, which includes our conscious awareness and emotional reactions to these sensory experiences, colored by memories of previous life experiences. Signals leaving the brain are not relayed through the thalamus.

HOW YOUR BODY MODULATES PAIN NATURALLY

Our complex and fascinating nervous system identifies and modulates pain through a system of electrical and chemical interaction. Neurons are the basic unit of the nervous system. They look like three-dimensional spiders with a central body and leglike projections that either receive from or transmit electrical messages to other cells. Most of the spider's legs, called dendrites, receive incoming nerve impulses. One of the legs, called the axon, can be more than two feet long. It is used to send impulses from the body to the spinal cord and up to the brain or from the brain down the spinal cord and out to the body.

Neurons allow us to respond to incoming information with appropriate movement and internal responses. For example, if we step on a nail, we perceive and react to the pain by quickly removing our foot from the source of pain (figures 1 and 2). The response to pain may also cause our heart to beat faster and our blood pressure to rise. We also learn to look for nails where we walk, having learned that they cause pain and are to be avoided. Like fireflies, neurons fire, or spontaneously produce electrical impulses on a regular basis—like a heartbeat. They may fire more or less slowly depending on whether they are excited or inhibited from firing by various types of chemicals called neurotransmitters.

Naturally occurring chemicals such as Substance P, glutamate, and

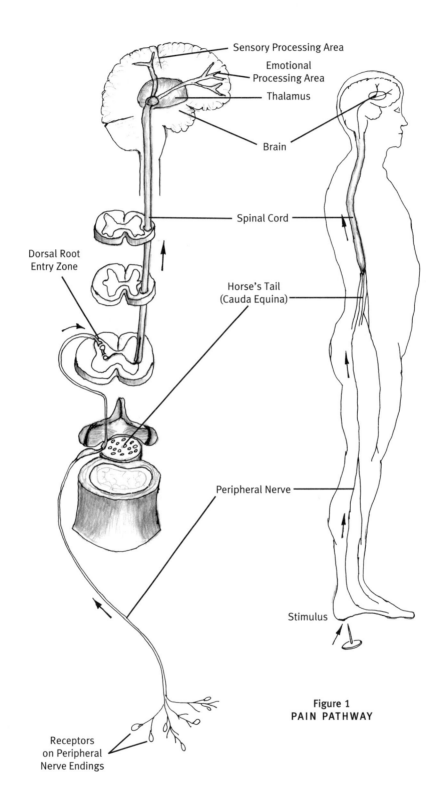

Sensory Processing Area

Emotional Processing Area

Thalamus

Brain

Spinal Cord

Dorsal Root Entry Zone

Horse's Tail (Cauda Equina)

Peripheral Nerve

Stimulus

Figure 1
PAIN PATHWAY

Receptors on Peripheral Nerve Endings

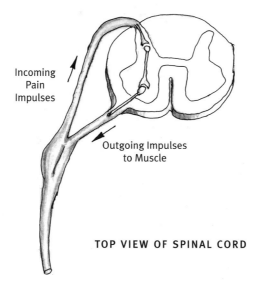

Incoming
Pain
Impulses

Outgoing Impulses
to Muscle

TOP VIEW OF SPINAL CORD

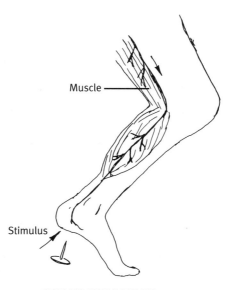

Muscle

Stimulus

REFLEX MECHANISM

Figure 2

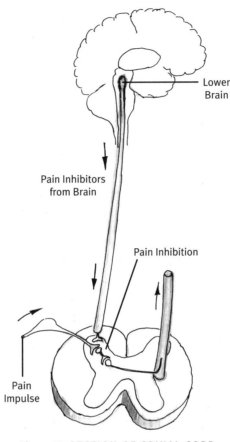

Lower
Brain

Pain Inhibitors
from Brain

Pain Inhibition

Pain
Impulse

Figure 3 SECTION OF SPINAL CORD

aspartate, excite neurons responsible for pain transmission. As you will see in chapter 3, drugs that block the action of these substances diminish our awareness of pain. Our body's narcoticlike chemicals, endorphins, and other substances in the brain and spinal cord inhibit the transmission of pain impulses.

Endorphins and other neurotransmitters with names such as GABA, serotonin, and norepinephrine are probably active in controlling pain when a wounded soldier runs through a battlefield with his arm blown to bits, unaware of the severity of the damage until someone stops him. (If we could only harness this on a daily basis!) Our own pain-relieving system appears to be activated by pain and stress, both of which affect the soldier, and even by suggestion or the placebo effect. Various drugs, discussed in chapter 3, enhance or mimic the effects of these inhibitory chemicals.

Nature has evolved two main central-nervous-system "wiring" strategies to reduce transmission of pain impulses from the spinal cord up to the brain (figure 3). Certain of the body's neurotransmitters can directly inhibit or slow down the activity of a pain-transmitting neuron. Or the nervous system can activate an inhibitory neuron to block the activity of the pain-transmitting cell. Both pain-reducing strategies are used simultaneously, resulting in fewer pain impulses reaching the brain. As a result, you feel better. Most pain-relieving drugs, and even some neurosurgical pain-relieving procedures, mimic or enhance these natural pain-relieving mechanisms.

The efficiency of this natural system of pain modulation may vary between individuals and between sexes. Some information suggests that premenopausal women have a greater tolerance for pain than men do. Could this create a survival advantage offsetting the transient disabilities of menstruation and childbirth? (Postmenopausal women have the same pain tolerance as men.) This may also partially explain personal differences in pain tolerance within the same sex. I say *partially* because cultural and psychological factors appear to be quite important in influencing pain tolerance as well—we'll get to that in a minute.

HOW WE THINK ABOUT AND FEEL PAIN

Different parts of the cortex, the covering of much of the brain, are responsible for conscious perception of pain sensations and how we process them intellectually and emotionally. The intellect processes the physical aspects of pain. You characterize the type of pain using intellectual constructs that describe the sensation (throbbing, burning) and locate it. If you have a small burn surrounded by an area of swelling and redness, you are aware that the surrounding inflamed skin is less tender than where the skin was actually burned. You become aware of what makes it feel better or worse.

The other part of pain processing is emotional—the interrelationship between your pain and your mood, and the effects of personality and culture on your reaction to pain. It involves areas of the brain distinct from those that process the pain intellectually, areas where your emotional reaction comes from—screaming in pain or simply becoming anxious about another suture being pulled. Emotionally, you perceive the unpleasant nature of the pain and how much of it you can stand.

Thankfully, we forget the intensity and quality of a painful act, whether it is witnessed and vividly imagined or personally experienced. This may have a definite survival value. Most women would never give birth to a second child if they could not forget about the pain of the first one. If we richly relived the full feelings associated with various painful experiences through which we have lived, directly or indirectly, we would hesitate to venture out of our beds in the morning. But we do forget.

Two elderly women on whom I had performed the same procedure within a month were in my office at the same time for a follow-up visit. Comparing notes, both women said the same thing, that although they were getting better, they felt as if they had been kicked by a horse. Well, as a rider, I have been kicked by a horse on occasion and thought we could discuss our experiences. I asked them when they had been around horses, and they both replied, "Never." They had never been kicked, but rightly or wrongly they surmised what such a blow must feel like and used that imagined feeling to describe their postoperative pain. In fact, neither of these women had ever been kicked by any animal bigger than their little brothers. Yet no doubt they had at least seen a horse kick its big, metal-covered hoof against a barn door with a loud bang. They must have mentally winced at the imagined pain such a kick could produce in a person, only to stuff this sharp pain out of consciousness. But it clearly wasn't forgotten. It came back to consciousness when the right trigger, the right kind of severe, bruiselike pain was experienced.

In the long run, with chronic pain, it is your conscious perception of pain and what it does that makes you anxious or depressed about it. Less predictable pain—like constant burning pain from a neuroma or scarred nerve—may be more psychologically debilitating than predictable pain that can be avoided by avoiding certain movements, like that associated with a sprained ankle, for example.

Pain does not always have to be described to be real, however. Infants, animals, and people who cannot speak express the impact of their pain with behavior such as grimacing, cringing, or changing posture. Until recently, it was assumed that children did not feel as much pain as adults did, and as a result, they often were not treated for pain.

VARIATIONS IN THE WAY WE PERCEIVE PAIN

A controlled three-second pulse of heat, held close to but never touching the skin, is described as painful by one of every two people. As the temperature increases, so does the sensation of pain. This suggests the evolution of a hardwired "danger point" in individuals with different personalities and across cultures—a universal perception of potentially tissue-damaging pain. The same sort of perception, at the same temperature range, is found in chimpanzees, baboons, and monkeys. A pain-sensing system is exceedingly important to survival and has been present in the animal kingdom since the evolution of the earliest fish and reptiles.

Depending on individual personality differences, which are a complicated product of genetic makeup, upbringing, and culture, we react to pain differently. Through complex connections within the brain, painful traumas are remembered and can provide the basis for learning from experience. (Falling out of a tree really hurts. I'll be careful next time to use good supporting branches.)

The frequency and severity of certain pain problems vary with cultures. In a study of male war veterans conducted in the early 1950s at the Mount Zion Hospital in San Francisco, Jews and Italians complained more freely of their pain than Anglo-Saxon Protestants or Irishmen. They all felt pain but reacted to it differently. As a resident at Bellevue Hospital in Manhattan I noticed that older Chinese immigrants appeared stoic about their pain. Whenever a Chinese patient appeared in the emergency room "in pain," I learned that what brought them there was often a severely painful condition. By the time I was a chief resident, I insisted that the staff working with me take this cultural stoicism into account in medicating these patients. Most of them needed narcotics and other painkillers, often in high doses, to alleviate pain. These patients also had serious medical or surgical conditions that required quick attention—like a tumor eroding the base of the skull, or a large herniated disk causing excruciating sciatica.

When the System Runs Amok: Sensitization

If water is dripped repeatedly on the same spot on your forehead, it will soon feel like a sledgehammer—the basis for an old form of torture. Understanding the process that leads to exaggerated responses to sensations is key to understanding disorders as disparate as fibromyalgia, a disease of sore muscles, and complex regional pain syndrome (CRPS), a form of neuropathic pain. Gently touch someone with either disorder and they will respond with anything from a wince to a howl and, in some cases, abruptly withdraw from your hand.

How do people in chronic pain develop excessive sensitivity to all sorts of stimulation, often covering large areas of their body that have never even been damaged? Through a process called sensitization, which stems from the abnormal processing of pain impulses. It results from continued stimulation, through injury or inflammation, of pain receptors in muscles and damaged peripheral nerves. Eventually the abnormal pain processing affects the spinal cord and brain.

If a peripheral nerve is repeatedly touched in a specific way, the repeated stimulation causes progressively greater sensitivity of peripheral pain receptors. These receptors become overreactive and send pain impulses to the spinal cord, out of proportion to their stimulation. In the water-torture example, if the dripping water is removed, the skin on the forehead will react normally again within a short period. In cases of prolonged peripheral painful stimulation, the neurons that carry pain impulses from the spinal cord to the brain also become sensitized. *The entire pain-processing system is out of order.*

Ongoing injury from a festering sore or muscle inflammation can cause supersensitivity. The continuing muscle soreness of fibromyalgia or a prolonged recovery from surgery may drive the pain-processing system into becoming progressively more sensitive. Any painful sensation, even a pinprick, may be perceived as excruciating, while something that normally does not hurt, like the stroke of a feather, may be perceived as painful. Like hyperactive children or adults, the sensitized nervous system can't quiet down quickly once it is activated. Once sensitization occurs, the abnormal response to various stimuli may become more widespread and difficult to control. Parts of the body that overreact in this manner may extend well beyond the original area of injury.

For example, sensitization may spread from the right ankle to a major part of the right leg. However, it can also spread to the left arm. This happens because a pain-transmitting neurotransmitter within the spinal cord, Substance P, can spread within the cord, from areas transmitting pain impulses from an injured right ankle to areas uninvolved with ankle sensation. This spread of Substance P then produces pain impulses corresponding to a noninjured area of the body—the left arm, for example. This spreading pain and sensitization is involved in many chronic pain states like fibromyalgia and CRPS.

Sensitization also spreads when new pain-propagating circuits grow within the central nervous system—a clear demonstration, by the way, that the spinal cord and brain do "grow" in adults. This means that the central nervous system has become a kind of free agent out on its own, transmitting pain impulses willy-nilly without obvious stimuli. This may explain why it is impossible to extinguish certain kinds of chronic pain once it has existed for a while, because it literally becomes a part of you.

Pain may spread by leaps and bounds, well beyond the nerves supplying the originally painful structure. This explains "total-body pain," which some physicians relatively unfamiliar with neuroscience label as psychiatric. You can understand why some chronic pain not only doesn't go away but gets worse with time, so it is absolutely essential to try to nip this process in the bud.

REFERRED PAIN: WHY THE CAUSE IS NOT ALWAYS NEAR THE EFFECT

Despite the wondrous nature of our nervous system, this incredibly complex and efficient living computer is not perfect. Pain impulses from several different sites in the body may converge on the same area within the spinal cord, which in turn sends information to the brain. Because of this overlap in the nervous system, we may perceive pain coming from a place that is not its actual source. This is known as referred pain.

For example, the heart and part of the left shoulder, arm, and fourth and fifth digits of the left hand send pain impulses to the same area of the spinal cord. If the heart becomes painful (angina), pain is often experienced in the left shoulder and arm. (Failure to understand this particular set of crossed pain signals has resulted in the death of people who had heart attacks but thought they had only a shoulder or arm problem.) The forehead and the upper spine both send pain impulses to the same area of the spinal cord. If parts of the upper spine are inflamed or damaged, the brain may erroneously interpret the pain as originating from the forehead. Irritation of the sacroiliac joint and the sciatic nerve may result in a similar confusion about the source of pain. At any spinal level, the disks, facets (joints supporting the spine), and nerve roots all feed pain information into the same level of the nervous system. All of these structures may cause a similar pattern of pain.

High-quality radiological studies, combined with a full history of the pain and a physical examination, may pinpoint the source of the problem. However, at times magnetic resonance imaging (MRI) or a

CAT scan will not explain the source of pain. It can be difficult to identify which structure is generating the pain, but it is not impossible. Knowledge of patterns of pain referred from various structures aids the physician in suggesting diagnoses that may not be obtainable by other means.

When there is no disk pressing on a nerve that would explain back and leg pain, proper evaluation of the facet joints, or even disks, which are *not* pressing on nerves in the lower spine, or of the sacroiliac joint, may elucidate the structure generating the pain. Diagnosis of these generators of pain is often aided by minimally invasive tests, such as nerve blocks (see chapter 7). Proper diagnosis is the most critical part of any pain-reduction therapy. The target in the spine must be identified and neutralized (made less painful) for the pain to cease. It is equally important to understand that if, after extensive evaluations by various professionals—don't ever stop at one—no correctable cause for the pain is found, it may be possible to relieve the pain with ongoing medication or other therapies.

TEST-NEGATIVE PAIN: WHEN THE CAUSE CAN'T BE SEEN

Imagine having severe, chronic pain over your eyebrow and a little neck pain, with a normal neurological and general physical examination. Is there something pressing on a nerve, or eroding the bone under the eyebrow—a slowly growing tumor, for example? Unfortunately, the MRI all too often reveals no abnormality, or at least not one that would explain the complaints. The pain may not even be related to a definite traumatic event like a whiplash injury or a well-understood systemic disease, like diabetes, known to produce pain. The condition is then considered to be test-negative. The pain has no objective basis—at least in terms of anatomical or physiological tests.

Test-negative painful conditions include:

- most headaches

- most muscle-related or myofascial pain

- certain nerve pains (neuralgias) in the head, face, and other body parts

- certain intermittent toothaches (often due to unseen cracks in tooth enamel that eventually break open)

- pain coming from the facets or joints supporting the spine

- possibly some pain due to diseased but not obviously herniated disks

The existence of so much uncertainty about who has pain and how much certainly underscores the inadequacy of our standard diagnostic tests. Paradoxically, the extraordinary success of modern medicine in extending life, correcting anatomical problems surgically, and demonstrating a myriad of disease processes—whether or not we can cure them all—has made it difficult for physicians to believe something exists if we cannot see it.

Without blood tests, X rays, and other diagnostic imaging techniques, physicians of past centuries were able to measure very little by today's standards. They had to rely on patient histories and physical examinations confined to the exterior of the body. Yet their extensive descriptions of disease indicate that they clearly believed in what they could not yet adequately see, touch, or measure.

Developing widely accepted tests to demonstrate and quantify pain is important. Such tests can remove the widespread frustration over the subjective nature of pain and measure results of treatment. Special MRI and nuclear medical techniques such as isotope-based positron emission tomography (PET) scans can study brain function. Some brain areas have higher or lower metabolism in various pain states, and this shows up visibly. These studies will be able to show us that a patient has pain, or depression, or both, in conditions with or without any apparent anatomical or physiological basis on X rays, regular MRIs, or other tests now used every day. These still-experimental studies of brain function could identify a physiological and biochemical basis for test-negative pain.

Research is under way to better determine which brain areas are involved in various pain states. The above types of radiological studies, which help delineate the function of various areas of the brain, may help us understand the mental and emotional aspects of pain that cannot be identified or are test-negative.

When not adequately treated in a timely fashion, patients with test-negative physical pain may develop significant secondary psychiatric symptoms. Physicians poorly schooled in the intricacies of appropriate diagnosis and treatment of test-negative painful conditions may actually help drive some patients with chronic pain syndromes to despair.

KEY POINTS
In Getting Your Pain Correctly Diagnosed

Your pain complaints should be taken seriously and evaluated using the conventional armamentarium, including a good history of the problem, a physical examination, and high-quality tests. When this standard evaluation, including radiological, physiological, and other conventional tests, is negative, or what appears abnormal on the office evaluation and laboratory tests doesn't fit your pain, you will be more likely to get a correct diagnosis if the following criteria are met:

- The doctor believes your pain is real.

- The doctor believes pain is a personal and subjective experience, colored by personality, personal history, and culture.

- The doctor knows the full range of pain syndromes and their causes.

- The doctor takes a full history and focuses on how this may relate to your current pain.

- The doctor performs a physical examination, focusing on the details of pain location, type of pain (burning, aching, throbbing, cramplike), and what makes it better or worse.

- The doctor employs, where appropriate, less conventional tests, such as diagnostic nerve blocks (see chapter 7) or other minimally invasive tests, and, in certain cases, even sophisticated imaging studies, to identify the source of the pain and understand how the pain is processed in the brain.

2

Controlling Pain Without Medication or Surgery

The value of life lies not in the length of days but in the use we make of them: a man may live long, yet get little from life. Whether you find satisfaction in life depends not on your tale of years, but on your will.

—MICHEL DE MONTAIGNE

Common sense and moderation sometimes appear to be antithetical to the fast pace of the information age. Yet they are the most important ingredients in any program designed to prevent pain. You are reading this book for one reason—you or someone you know is in pain and you want to know what can be done about it. Before we discuss medical treatments, let's see if you are causing yourself pain with poor posture or sleep positions, or by the way you work or play.

Lowering the risk of developing an illness implies an attempt to prevent it. Prevention involves work, and work involves discipline. You have to decide how you want to take care of the body you live in— and try to assure it as long a drive as possible without a breakdown. That means making choices and paying attention to things that you never thought about as a youngster. In a way, the older you get, the more discipline you must have, not less. At a certain point in life, true discipline involves learning to burn the candle only at one end—making those lifestyle changes that reduce both the mental pressure and the physical stress of life.

LIFESTYLE CHANGES

Although our lives have evolved to make us more sedentary, our bodies have not adjusted to the change. Humans were not designed to sit for extended periods of time. Get up and move periodically. When you sit, use a chair that offers back support. The Gothic church chair is better for your back than all of these high-tech ergonomic extravaganzas that we claim to be comfortable. Of course, people in medieval Europe had enough sense—or little enough heat—that they did not sit for sixteen hours at a time.

Warm up before any physical activity, even regular ones. Warm-ups mean that little by little the heart rate goes up and muscles get more blood. All muscles, tendons, and ligaments must be stretched. One of my patients is a garbage collector who gets up early. On winter mornings he makes his rounds seated in a warm truck, but periodically he must step outside into the cold, abruptly lifting large, heavy cans without any warm-up preparation. One morning, he arose quickly from the bent position to lift a heavy can and injured some of the coverings of the joints and disks that support his lower back, causing excruciating pain and laying him up for several weeks. I would like to recommend to the Department of Sanitation that workers start their day by doing warm-up exercises followed by some calisthenics.

In developing nations like India, workers carry heavy loads on their backs (or even heads), but they sing or chant while they work. This gives them a rhythm to work to, so they are slow and regular in their movements, not quick or jerky. Sudden lifting, or any sudden movement, is what gets us into trouble. In this country, a law associate sits for twelve hours a day and then rushes to get in a two-hour squash game—without warming up or mentally and physically relaxing before the game. A great prescription for developing back and other problems. A manual laborer in India, despite his physically hard life, may have a healthier back.

Doctors who treat spinal and related disorders deal with the medical backlash from a demanding workplace. Many disabilities come from people doing more than they should, whether it is too much physical exertion in otherwise out-of-shape individuals or spending too many hours at their desks without moving. Society objectifies the self. We objectify ourselves. We treat new cars better than we treat ourselves.

You will work longer and harder and more productively if you take time to be fit. During the more complicated pain-relieving surgical procedures I perform, I may stand for two to three hours at a time in one place. We are not meant to do this. If you stand a lot, as I do, shift from hip to hip to avoid bursitis and back pain. Don't be a weekend athletic warrior or think you're going to redesign your own garden along the lines of Versailles in one weekend.

Athletics and gardening are pleasures of life. Anyone—urbanite, suburbanite, or even rural dweller—needs such activities. Moderation is key. Warm up, even before weeding. Someone who exercises every day is less likely to get hurt than someone who does it only on weekends. Dragging fifty pounds of peat moss on the weekend after spending your week at a desk can precipitate a tear or significant strain in the supporting structures of your back. No matter what you do for a living, your body is your instrument, for yourself and for your family. Take care of it. It can't always be fixed to be as good as new. And you can't turn it in for a new one when the lease runs out or when the repairs have become prohibitive. Here are some commonsense rules.

- Warm up.

- Relax your back.

- Change your posture.

- Keep your weight down. (A paunch will make your back as well as your abdomen weak.)

- Start an exercise program to keep back muscles limber and well tuned.

- Lift large or heavy objects with your whole body by bending at the knees.

- Adults carrying little children on their shoulders risk cervical (the medical term for *neck*) disk herniation in that forward-bent neck.

- Extreme arching of your neck, such as doing back flips, can also herniate disks.

- If you have an ache or pain, find out what's wrong.

- Don't run on a sore Achilles tendon.

- When carrying heavy or awkward objects, divide them between your arms. Don't carry things on just one side of your body. In Manhattan, where I work, most people don't have cars and they lug an outrageous number of things at once in shoulder bags or backpacks and in the crook of their arms.

- Try a kneeler chair to see if it relieves back pain.

- Straight-backed chairs are better than deep ones that don't support your back.

- When driving a car, sit as upright as possible.

Position Your Resting Body

The back is injured most frequently in the daytime, when excessive weight or strain is applied to it. In contrast, the neck is most often injured during sleep, when one tosses and turns, which twists the disks of the neck. Many cervical-disk herniations are noted as you awaken, not as you try to lift something. I'm not sure how effectively a cervical-disk herniation can be prevented by proper nighttime positioning, but a few ideas come to mind. I do believe your nighttime position influences your pain and overall recovery—or lack thereof—from a cervical-disk herniation.

People often ask me what kind of mattress they should have. I reply quite honestly that I don't know and I don't think anyone else does either. Get a mattress that you—and your other half, if there is one—likes. Does a "good mattress" improve your spine? I'm not sure it can alter your anatomy, but it certainly can give you a better night's sleep and make you feel better. The more you toss and turn, the worse it is for your neck.

If you have neck problems, make the effort to sleep on your back, even though it is hard to do. Pillows are important. Use a good pillow that is soft enough to keep your neck from arching severely but large and hard enough to raise your head slightly at your shoulder level. For those with neck pain, I am not convinced cervical pillows are a good means of relieving neck pain for all people. By all means, if you have one and feel it helps you, use it. However, many of these "therapeutic pillows," like traveling pillows, may make you arch your neck and put more pressure on the disks and facets (joints stabilizing the spine; see figure 7). This could worsen some painful conditions affecting the neck.

The Body at Play

The athletic prowess that many middle-aged people developed in their youth may now cause a lifestyle dilemma. These people may have the mind-set and even the ability to ski a double-black-diamond slope, even in bad conditions, at forty miles per hour or more. But their bodies may not be as forgiving as they were in youth—especially the bodies of weekend or ski-vacation athletes. Have you ever noticed how elegantly older ski instructors ski, even down those demanding slopes? Many excellent younger skiers may pass them, but so what? The trick is to do it enjoyably and well, but carefully enough to be able to keep on doing it, whether your livelihood depends on it or not. Remember common sense and moderation.

As you age, you may wish to reduce your level of performance so you can perform longer. Decide if injuring yourself is worth winning—or, more likely, finishing—a race. Yes, I know about the runner's high, those wonderful endorphins—your body's own narcotics. Thank God they're not regulated. Marathons would take days instead of hours!

Highly competitive, rough sports; pounding sports; or potentially dangerous sports (horseback riding, mountain climbing, gymnastics, skydiving, to name a few) can be psychologically and physically rewarding, but all can cause lifelong painful injuries. However, regular moderate exercise is a safe, beneficial, and, I believe, even necessary component to a life of vitality and vigor. President Kennedy was right in emphasizing a national physical-fitness program. Properly applied, it provided a formula for physical and mental fitness—and for keeping Americans thin. Unfortunately, on one hand, the formula is not followed by enough of us, and on the other, it may have started the exercise craze to which some of us are still attracted, often with injurious effects. If only Americans didn't always have to do everything as a craze, but could do things in moderation. Maybe my wish for moderation defies the can-do attitude that made this country great. Fine, but just a little moderation, especially as we get older, may help reduce painful wear and tear. (In chapter 8 I will discuss preventing and treating painful sports injuries.)

I used to be a long-distance runner, have climbed extensively (major technical climbs to about twenty-three thousand feet), actively ride and even jump horses, and enjoy skiing (when global warming gives me a break), but I am aware that what I am doing may cause pain or disability. I try to be careful and always warm up and stretch before athletics and cool down afterward. If I haven't exercised in a while because of travel, work, or illness, I start up again slowly. I try to keep my weight within a five-pound range, and that is not always easy as I get older and am more sedentary than when I was younger. I never snack. I eat a high-quality Mediterranean diet, including occasional meat and sweets, and drink alcohol (mostly red wine) in moderation.

I never eat less than two hours before bedtime. I also smoke an occasional cigar or pipe. This regime works well for me. It works well for most of the people in Europe, where I was raised. I am not holding myself up, by any means, as a model to emulate. I do represent a typical person who may have pain.

I gave up expedition-style mountain climbing for one reason and one reason alone. The summer of the year before I was planning to climb Mount Denali in Alaska, I awoke one morning with a damaged disk in my neck pressing on a nerve going into my left arm, causing pain, numbness, and weakness. I got better without surgery. The disk shrank to some extent. But it took several months. I took steroids by mouth, which treated my left arm problems, but made me a bit "crazy," and I also used a collar and special pillow to sleep. I had two closed MRIs—in spite of some claustrophobia. However, to this day, if I overdo it with that arm, or carry heavy loads for a long time, or don't sleep quite right, I feel some pain in my shoulder or arm. It always gets better, but I'm careful. I can't afford to take part in a major climb and have to bail out, letting my fellow climbers or myself down, because of that disk declaring itself horribly at an inopportune moment, two-thirds of the way up a major peak.

While Traveling

We all travel more than ever before. It can be fun, work, or hell, depending on how you do it and how much pain you are in, or develop, as a result of doing it. I do think some precautions may limit travel-related pain.

On planes, trains, and buses, sit on an aisle where you can move more easily. If you have a bad back and fly coach, try to reserve the first seat at the bulkhead, or on the exit rows, where you have more leg room. Sitting up straight during the flight is usually preferable for low-back-pain sufferers. If you have neck problems and are taking a long flight, decide for yourself if a cervical traveling pillow is good for you as you travel. Use of such devices is a function of what's comfortable, not what your doctor says.

If you travel frequently, get a credit card and join a frequent-flyer program that gives you access to an airport lounge where you can relax in a good chair.

Someone with a bad neck or bad back should distribute the weight of what he or she carries rather than tote everything in one hand. (See how many people in airports carry two suitcases in one hand and a two-ounce ticket in the other.)

Don't store heavy objects in overhead racks. Carefully put them on the floor under your seat to avoid the strain of reaching up to pull down an awkward weight. Pick up your baggage carefully as well. Ask for help from the flight attendants, if needed. Don't carry a heavy garment bag that you must store in the overhead rack.

When reserving plane seats in coach class, ask for flights that are not completely booked so that you can stretch out in the empty seats. Book your flight well in advance and get the best seat.

If you take a two-week trip somewhere, consider whether traveling in coach, where you'll be squashed for hours, is really worth the savings, considerable though they may be. It may pay to book a roomier but more expensive seat that will protect your back so you can enjoy your two-week vacation and then return to work so you can pay for it.

Spend money on accommodations with a decent bed that will protect your back and enable you to enjoy your vacation.

If you have neck and/or back pain, someone must help with your baggage. Look for a porter to help you rather than relying on your spouse or significant other, because they can wear out too.

Tip the cabdriver or van driver explicitly to help you with your luggage. Do not try to be macho, and this goes for women as well as men.

If you rent a car, check the model to make sure it is comfortable for you and easy to load and unload—just in case you are in a pickle in a small Tuscan town and nobody is around to unload your baggage. Some small rental cars can be bad for you.

Driving and not knowing where you are going is stressful. Nervous tension makes pain worse and the body more disposed to break down.

Know where you're going and how to get there. Plan ahead.

Wear comfortable shoes, suitable to what you are doing. If you are walking for hours through unpaved paths in the countryside or on cobblestone streets, you will want some form of excellent walking shoe or even a light hiking shoe. Heavy hiking shoes would be overkill.

If you carry heavy equipment, such as cameras, balance it on your body—as you did with your luggage. Special vests for photographers may be helpful.

Fanny belts, not the majority of packs poorly designed for carrying heavy weight, are the best solution for carrying weight for a long period of time.

Even when you are shopping for souvenirs, balance packages in your two arms. Don't walk around hunched over to the front or to one side.

If you have physical problems, take along all the medicines you use, including pain medication. Be careful about drinking alcohol if you are taking pain medicine. I didn't say avoid the wonderful local wine, but realize it may interact with your medicine to make you sleepy. Nonsteroidal medications (NSAIDs; see chapter 3) like aspirin, ibuprofen (Motrin, Advil), or naprosyn (Aleve) combined with alcohol are more likely to irritate your stomach.

Think ahead to be up to physical demands. If you know walking causes pain in your low back and you want to visit a museum, take pain medications forty-five minutes before you anticipate needing it, so it is already in your body before the pain begins. It works better that way. Don't just pop a pill in your mouth when pain hits—it won't work very well if you do.

Take extra care to follow the dosing schedules of your medication. Most medications last only three to four hours. If you need lots of pain medicine, reconsider your activities and adjust gradually to the pace of wherever you are, allowing for changing time zones.

Depending on your medical history and where you are going, you may want to bring medicine for coughing, constipation, and vomiting. These problems can cause disk-related pain or make it worse.

Changing times zones can affect your sleep. Organize the first day or two of activities to ease into the new time zone. You may have to stay up later the day of arrival to get into the sleep pattern of the place to which you have traveled.

On vacation, many people deny they are in pain until they can't stand it. When it gets to that point, you have ruined the day—and possibly a few more. All the medicine you can get your hands on still might not turn you around quickly enough. Be vigilant and nip pain in the bud with medication and lifestyle changes.

If you get off the plane and your back hurts, rest, no matter what! If you have a bad back, consider a beach vacation that offers warmth and water.

Don't drink alcohol and coffee on the flight. These will impair your sleep and exacerbate jet lag, which, in turn, could further impair your sleep and normal daytime activity and make your pain worse.

Pace yourself. When you're fatigued and irritable you're likely to experience pain.

Watching Your Weight

Increasingly Americans are overweight, according to various medical studies. This has been happening gradually over the past few decades because we not only eat more and differently but move less. We used to eat three meals a day and do more physical work. Now we eat all the time, not only at home but in the shopping mall, at the movies, at the ball game. We also eat fast foods high in fat, starch, and sugar. Our work has become less physical and we spend the day in front of a computer and go home and flop on the couch. Being overweight becomes a chronic disease from which it gets more and more difficult to recover the longer you have it. It also contributes to an enormous number of medical problems, including heart disease and diabetes.

Excess weight wears out your musculoskeletal system prematurely, causing an accelerated risk of disk herniation and spinal slippage. Both of these conditions lead to surgery, and potentially repeated surgery in the overweight patient, in whom these problems are more likely to recur. Overweight people are more likely to have problems with weight-bearing joints, leading to joint-replacement surgery. Once they are replaced, the artificial joints wear out and the process has to be repeated every ten to twenty years or so. (Artificial hips last longer and cause less pain than artificial knees.) Before, during, and just after these surgeries, you will suffer from some degree of pain.

So, by eating poorly and being sedentary you will become married to the medical system, and it'll be a bad marriage, especially for you. Excess weight also places a greater burden on your heart, blood vessels, and metabolic system, inviting atherosclerosis (hardening and clogging of blood vessels) and diabetes. Associated with one or both of these conditions are high blood pressure, heart failure and attacks, stroke, kidney disease and dialysis, visual loss, and damage to the peripheral nerves (neuropathy; see chapter 7). Neuropathy, in turn, results in numbness, weakness, pain, impotence, and digestive-system disturbance. Eating late at night helps accumulate excess weight, and this eating pattern is often associated with dysfunction of the stomach and esophagus—the tube connecting the mouth to the stomach. This may lead to cancer of the esophagus and death.

NONMEDICAL PAIN MANAGEMENT

I have pain patients who ask what besides medicine and surgery can relieve their pain. Even if you take proper pain medication, or consider

other treatments such as invasive pain management or surgery, you or
your doctor may want to investigate physical therapy, behavioral therapy, various pain-relieving devices, and alternative or complementary
medicine. Most of my patients have seen several physicians and tried
various kinds of treatments, including those below, before coming to
me—still in pain. Therefore, I personally have little chance to "order"
the therapies below. Nevertheless, I can discuss the therapeutic roles
they may and may not have.

Physical Therapy

Physical or occupational therapy can do many wonderful things in the
right setting. It may help someone who is stiff or out of shape, from
chronic pain or from wearing a cast, become limber. It can recondition
people who have lost the ability to walk because of a severe accident,
a stroke, or an amputation. Even if patients need the help of canes,
crutches, or walkers, they learn how to use the devices made to maximize their function. Such therapy helps them tone up and learn to use
their bodies properly again so they don't harm themselves walking
with their impairment.

Physical therapy doesn't heal the nerves or muscles weakened by
stroke, accident, or surgery. It "teaches" new coordination and new
uses for the remaining, intact nerves and muscles to compensate for
whatever was lost. When you have a knee replacement, you learn to
bend the new knee through the pain of the scars and incisions, eventually learning to walk as if you were using your original knee before
it became damaged. For all these things, physical therapy is very effective. However, for the relief or control of severe chronic pain caused
by nerve damage or compression, I do not think it is effective. Physical therapy is not likely to be tolerated—or effective—in treating the
severe pain and disability resulting from a large disk herniation. Analgesics, activity as tolerated, and, if needed, surgery should be used in
these cases.

If you have severe lumbar stenosis, a narrowing of the spinal canal,
that causes painful pressure on the nerves, physical therapy is not a
good use of your resources or time. You probably need surgery. Indeed,
the best time to spend your annual Medicare allotment for in-patient
physical therapy is after, not before, surgery. Then it can help build up
muscles that became weak before surgery. Unfortunately, it is often
used inappropriately and unsuccessfully as a substitute for surgery.

I recommend physical therapy for patients in chronic pain, who are stiff or weak following surgery or other trauma, stroke, or osteo-porotic fractures. It can also help a stiff or "frozen" shoulder follow-ing a prolonged bout of neck and arm pain due to a cervical disk herniation. A "frozen" shoulder may cause pain and disability long after the cervical disk has healed. Physical therapy must be accompa-nied by appropriate pain control, through whatever means, for the pa-tient to be able to participate fully in his or her rehabilitation.

Can physical therapy hurt a patient? Usually not in the long run, al-though it may cause some pain. Some people feel better in the physi-cal therapist's office, but when they go home the pain comes back. If physical therapy has not given you significant ongoing relief after two months of treatment, you may be wasting your time and money.

The type of physical treatment that is best for you is best decided by a physiatrist, a physician specially trained in physical medicine. They are the best qualified to issue instructions to physical therapists. I so strongly believe in this that I almost always send patients to physia-trists for physical-therapy evaluation and, as a rule, will not direct the activities of physical therapists myself.

The Relaxation Response

The human relaxation response, which was popularized by Dr. Her-bert Benson, has been used quite successfully to treat various kinds of pain. The response is often subjectively experienced as a sense of well-being, peace of mind, and feeling at ease with the world. All of these constitute an altered state of consciousness. This method slows down your breathing, lowers your blood pressure, relaxes your muscles, and changes your brain-wave activity. This response is the opposite of the fight-or-flight response associated with fear or an emergency situation, including severe, acute pain. There are a variety of techniques to reach this state, but ultimately, in the state, you relax. Often repetition of a word or sound, known as a mantra, helps. Transcendental meditation is one technique for achieving this response.

An important feature of the relaxation response is its prolonged benefit, which far outlasts the actual relaxing mental exercise. It ap-pears that pain is perceived differently under the influence of this re-sponse. Pain impulses are still transmitted (body) but are perceived with less suffering (mind). It is as if the alarm reaction of the mind is somehow deconditioned and no longer responds with the same mag-nitude when confronted by bodily pain. The relaxation response can give you some relief and sense of mastery over your condition.

Hypnosis

Hypnosis and even self-hypnosis may help alleviate painful conditions in some people. It has been used successfully for cancer pain, in dentistry, with burn patients, with children undergoing minor painful procedures, and in obstetrics. Hypnosis can be used to give direct suggestions for pain relief or as an adjunct to psychotherapy or other behavioral treatment.

Unfortunately, not everyone is readily hypnotized, and the best results from using hypnosis to control pain are achieved in patients who are easily hypnotized.

Hypnosis also produces a relaxation response, as well as phenomena unique to hypnosis. These include possible distorted perceptions, a sense of going back in time, forgetfulness about what happened during the hypnotic episode, and the ability by the hypnotist to suggest a course of action to be followed by the subject following hypnosis.

In other words, hypnosis is not just a form of relaxation response. The mechanism underlying hypnosis is not entirely clear, but it can be effective in certain patients and belongs in the pain-management toolbox.

Biofeedback

We can learn to control our brain-wave activity; to raise or lower our pulse and blood pressure; to increase blood supply to one area, such as an arm, with a resultant warming of that hand compared with the other; and to relax muscles. Biofeedback helps us modify autonomic-nervous-system responses. This is the part of the nervous system that automatically controls our minute-to-minute physiology, such as heartbeat and blood pressure, without our awareness. Biofeedback provides feedback on these otherwise unconscious biological processes with the goal of giving us control over them. With the help of a trained technician you are hooked up to electronic instruments that monitor your muscle tension, skin temperature, pulse, and brain-wave activity. You can learn to voluntarily control the process, including some that involve pain.

Biofeedback is based on the relaxation response and the work of B. F. Skinner, who refined the concept that animals could be taught to control behavior based on a system of rewards. Biofeedback has been touted as a way to help many people relax sore muscles and get prolonged benefit in the treatment of recurring tension headaches, migraines, and myofascial pain (a form of muscle pain), to name a few conditions (see chapters 4 and 5).

A woman who suffered from tension headaches due to tight muscles over her skull tried biofeedback. A technician put a device over her head and told her to keep the light on the attached machine green. When the woman's scalp muscles were relaxed, the light was green. If they tightened, the light became red. The woman seemingly could learn to use her mind to control her body. Actually, her body learned to control itself. Although paying attention is important for learning through biofeedback, too much focus on the details of the biofeedback training can be counterproductive.

By paying attention to the lights, or other types of feedback from various machines, the woman "learned" to keep her scalp and neck muscles relaxed. Once this method is learned, it can continue without the machine, which is the obvious objective. When those who learn to use this method feel a headache coming on, they use what they have learned in biofeedback sessions to control the muscles or the blood vessels that contribute to the headache. Biofeedback requires trial, error, and a lot of practice.

Biofeedback appears to be best used in conjunction with other techniques for attaining relaxation, like relaxation-response training and hypnosis. For those whom these techniques help, the investment of time and money is more than worth it. When they work, they give people control over their pain without medication or with the need for less medication.

TENS

Transcutaneous electrical nerve stimulation, or TENS, is the use of electrical impulses, delivered at a range of intensities, lengths of impulse, and frequencies of impulse, applied to the skin through small EKG-like electrodes, for the relief of pain. While it is not a cure for pain, it may relieve symptoms in some patients. Some studies suggest it may relieve up to half the pain in more than half the patients. According to others, it has no long-term benefit in the treatment of low-back pain (see chapter 6).

The impulses are delivered by a battery-powered device about the size of a pack of cards that you can attach to your belt. Slim wires run from the unit to electrodes placed on your skin around the painful areas of your body or on areas lying within the same distribution of the spinal nerves that receive sensation from the painful area. The location of the electrodes is determined both by knowledge of the pathways through which pain signals reach the spinal cord from the periphery and empirically, by trial and error.

You can activate the TENS unit at will. In one frequently used method of TENS stimulation, the unit is activated for a few minutes every hour and repeated as needed. The unit can also be kept on nearly continuously, with breaks as short as three minutes between stimulation. TENS feels like a mix of mild tingling and strong pins-and-needles sensations, and certain settings of the machine may produce muscle contractions, depending on the intensity of stimulation. By increasing the intensity and length of the impulses, the stimulation spreads and deepens. Optimal response guides the most efficient setting.

TENS achieves pain reduction by using one kind of stimulation to diminish the processing of pain impulses. It has an effect on pain similar to that obtained by biting, licking, or rubbing a burned or banged finger. The stimulation activates nerves that compete with and inhibit the processing of incoming pain impulses at the level of the spinal cord. TENS also increases the level of endorphins, our own naturally occurring narcotics, which inhibit pain impulses from rising to the brain from the spinal cord. Some studies indicate it may affect the autonomic nervous system as well. TENS is often used for the relief of various types of acute and chronic pain, including:

- musculoskeletal pain

- neuropathic pain

- pain due to insufficient blood supply

- cancer pain

- abdominal and pelvic pain due to menstrual cramps and various painful bladder problems

- certain kinds of head and facial pain (headaches and temporo-mandibular-joint-related pain, for example)

- postoperative pain

This treatment is not a cure, but TENS may diminish painful symptoms and give you a sense of control over your pain and treatment. However, TENS is best used in conjunction with other therapy such as medication, physical therapy, acupuncture, and psychological therapy. Many of my patients have used TENS with some benefit, but not many of them have been satisfied with it for extended periods of time.

Nevertheless, those who have purchased a TENS device usually feel the purchase was worthwhile.

No adverse effects of TENS have been documented. However, as a precaution, TENS should not be used if you have a pacemaker. It is not meant to be worn over the carotid arteries (in the neck), near the eyes, or over the front of the chest (especially if you have heart problems). It should be used with caution if you are pregnant.

I have an arrangement with TENS manufacturers, so TENS units may be given to patients on a free trial basis, and if they find it effective, they buy it from the supplier. I review the optimal electrode placements and device settings with my patient and we come up with one or even a few settings that appear to help their pain. They then take the unit home and experiment for one to two weeks before deciding on purchasing such a device from a company. Without proper instructions or a trial period, a patient cannot really tell if the device is appropriate for his or her condition.

Frequently, patients are given TENS treatments during physical-therapy sessions, with a maximum of six hours of pain relief, but are not given a unit for home use. Obviously, such a policy makes little sense for the patient who may come in for therapy two to three times weekly.

Psychological Therapy
Another noninterventional treatment on the lower rungs of the pain-management ladder is psychotherapy or behavior therapy. The way you deal psychologically with pain can make you feel like a down-trodden victim, a tough resistance fighter, or something in between. Your approach to dealing with pain may include making a truce with aspects of pain and the limitations it imposes on your functional existence. In the worst case, chronic pain can make you look at life through glasses tinted with fiery red pain or even black melancholy.

One of the things a good psychotherapist can do is give you strategies to cope with the pain, given who you are, how you were raised, and your own earlier experiences with pain. If your grandmother lived with you toward the end of her life, chronically disabled with painful rheumatoid arthritis, your knowledge of what she went through can cause you to experience your own pain with more fear and pessimism than someone brought up in an athletic, gregarious, cheerful family. A chronically anxious or depressed person will cope poorly with chronic pain. He or she is more likely to spiral downward psychologically, so-

cially, and economically if pain causes a cessation of activities that
help a person achieve sound mental health. Chronic pain breeds anxiety and depression and is the basis of a vicious cycle.

Psychotherapeutic techniques have changed significantly over the last
two generations, resulting in a more focused, problem-oriented approach. Rather than spending indeterminate lengths of time analyzing
the influence of childhood events on a patient's difficulty in coping with
his or her pain, many contemporary therapists help patients to focus on
their pain, problems related to it, and psychological and practical
lifestyle strategies of dealing with the pain and related problems. Skilled
direction from the therapist and strong commitment from the patient
can isolate the "mind" contribution to a pain problem, and progress can
be made in moderating its devastating power to overwhelm the patient
emotionally, socially, economically, and even spiritually.

Psychiatrists or psychotherapists skilled at dealing with people in
physical pain will focus on practical day-to-day solutions tailored to
the individual pain patient. Obviously, these recommendations must
take into account past as well as present problems, and ongoing psychotherapy should provide strategies for coping with pain and disability and deciding on and implementing lifestyle changes to reduce
pain. For example, learning to modify or give up an activity to gain
pain relief may also allow you to get involved in a satisfying replacement activity. Since pain causes depression and anxiety and both of
these can increase perceived pain, it can also be useful to take antidepressants and other psychiatric medication as part of the comprehensive treatment. Enlisting a psychiatrist who is trained in dealing with
patients suffering from chronic pain will also provide access to any
necessary psychiatric medication. Physicians who are not psychiatrists
should not treat depression or anxiety except in special situations such
as lack of access to specialists.

Psychiatrists are specialists who are most familiar with psychiatric
medications and their side effects and interactions with other drugs.
They also may use psychotherapy and/or behavior modification with
patients. Psychiatrists are usually far more skilled at these therapeutic
techniques than any other type of physician.

If a patient does not need psychiatric medication, other options
exist, such as licensed psychologists or social workers trained in psychotherapy who have experience in dealing with pain. However, fragmented care may lead to therapeutic conflicts and logistical difficulties.

When someone says, "I see the psychiatrist for medication, the psychologist for my psychotherapy, the pain specialist for narcotics and other pain medication, the neurologist for the evaluation of my disk herniation, and the gastroenterologist for management of my narcotic-induced constipation," then the use of specialists has reached absurd, counterproductive proportions.

ALTERNATIVE AND COMPLEMENTARY MEDICINE

Americans spend approximately $27 billion a year on herbal remedies, chiropractors, and massage therapists. In the 1990s, as the popularity of alternative medicine grew and as the cost of traditional or allopathic medicine soared, the National Institutes of Health began funding studies that would provide the public with useful information regarding the efficacy of treatment other than traditional medicine. In 1998, the *Journal of the American Medical Association* published studies identifying some treatments that seemed to work and others that were ineffective. However, little is now known about the safety, efficacy, and cost-effectiveness of alternative procedures for most conditions and about why and how they work.

The public uses alternative, or complementary, therapy for a variety of reasons. Obviously, if Western medicine had all the answers, no other therapy would be sought and used. For many users of alternative/complementary medicine, Western medical therapy may be viewed as ineffective and expensive depending on their experience with the system or doctors. However, before seeking alternative care, consider the facts. Using the scientific method, Western medicine has developed the most effective treatments for most of the afflictions of mankind, including the most potentially serious. For any condition, whatever its level of gravity, when Western medicine has proven to be either effective but costly or associated with severe side effects, or just ineffective, alternative treatments must be entertained, including those arising from a non-Western medical system. However, regardless of the type of treatment, all therapy should be evaluated scientifically. Ineffective treatment of any kind should be abandoned.

Many of the patients who see me long ago failed to derive adequate pain relief from treatments like physical therapy, TENS, relaxation-related techniques, psychotherapy, and alternative or complementary treatments like glucosamine, chiropractic manipulation, massage, herbal remedies, and acupuncture. These therapies may have a role at various stages of chronic pain, especially in situations where the pain is not severe or is at least partially controlled by other means.

The potential harm of some alternative therapy results from the fact that approximately 70 percent of patients who use alternative medicine *do not tell their physicians that they are doing so*. If no one knows how alternative medicines work, then certainly no one knows how they interact with Western therapies. Just because a treatment is alternative and can be obtained without a prescription doesn't mean it is innocuous. For example, the herb Saint-John's-wort may result in serious complications during anesthesia if the anesthesiologist uses certain drugs.

The American Society of Anesthesiologists and the New York Society of Anesthesiologists have warned patients to stop taking herbal medicines two to three weeks before scheduled operations. They recommend that patients advise doctors of what they are taking, or show them the containers, if they cannot go off the drugs in that period. Aside from this, if my patients find that alternative medicine and therapies work for them, I am happy for them—as long as there are no untoward side effects from the treatment.

Acupuncture

Acupuncture is a therapeutic process in which specific points of the body are stimulated with needles to foster healing or pain relief. The theory is that there are two thousand points in the body connecting twenty meridians, or pathways of energy. Stimulating these points restores health to the mind and body by balancing a person's energy. Western researchers theorize that in cases where acupuncture eases pain, it does so by stimulating the central nervous system to release chemicals that lessen the perception of pain.

However it works, acupuncture has a role in management of short-term acute pain and seems to have some benefit for the treatment of certain chronic pain problems such as headaches, bursitis, arthritic joints, and muscle strain. To date, there is insufficient data supporting the use of acupuncture in treating chronic pain. In the long run, the role of acupuncture and other traditional and nontraditional pain-control methods has to be determined through outcome studies. These questions must be asked and answered: How effective is the treatment and for how long? What are the costs and risks? How does it compare to other treatments for the same problem?

The Federal Food and Drug Administration estimates that nine to twelve million patients spend as much as five hundred million dollars on acupuncture treatments per year. In the year 2000, an estimated twenty thousand licensed acupuncturists were practicing in thirty-four states and the District of Columbia. In 1999, more than three thousand medical doctors trained in acupuncture were practicing in all fifty states.

In some cases of musculoskeletal pain or headache, I have sent patients to acupuncturists, usually after the patients have asked me about the treatment. It was evident, however, that few found sustained relief. My own observations are echoed in a recent medical report in *Spine* that surveyed various studies of the effect of acupuncture on low-back pain. The results were decidedly negative. Of eleven studies, only two were of high scientific quality and these showed no benefit of acupuncture over treatments such as TENS or trigger-point injections. It is important, however, for patients to exhaust all forms of treatment before progressing to more costly and serious interventions. Since at least a modest percentage of patients with chronic lumbar-spine pain from arthritis or trauma improved somewhat during a course of acupuncture treatment, this alternative treatment deserves our attention.

Laser Energy to the Skin
A newer technique, which delivers laser energy to the skin overlying painful areas of the body, was applied to low-back-pain sufferers in a well-controlled study. The technique resulted in moderate short-term benefit, with the effect of treatment wearing off in one month.

Spinal Manipulation
Chiropractic manipulation has been the subject of studies and stories that offer a conflicting picture as to whether or not this means of treatment is beneficial. Responding to this situation and aware of the popularity of chiropractic, the National Institutes of Health have funded studies to look into its effectiveness. What little research that has been published thus far indicates that physical manipulation of sore, tight body parts does make people feel better. My own opinion is a guarded one, especially when it involves treatment for head, neck, and shoulder pain.

Various, somewhat confusing, data indicate that chiropractic manipulation is effective for treating acute low-back pain, with or without neurological involvement or "sciatica." The Agency for Health

Care Policy and Research, part of the U.S. Department of Health and Human Services, has stated that spinal manipulation hastens recovery from acute low-back pain and has advised against lower-back surgery except in the most severe cases.

One reason chiropractic manipulation makes people feel better is the benefit of being touched therapeutically. According to a study of 321 adults with only low-back pain (without sciatica), reading a booklet about back pain was about as effective as chiropractic manipulation or physical therapy in treating low-back pain. However, 70 percent of the participants who had experienced the two physically oriented therapies were happy with their treatment versus only 30 percent of people who had done nothing but read the booklet without seeing a practitioner. Reading is far less expensive and more convenient than visiting an office, but people would rather have someone listen to them and be physically touched by a health professional. "Laying on of hands" is an intrinsic part of the healing process—something that is not readily dealt with in the "human widget-processing" health-care system under which so many patients and physicians live for the moment.

The differences between the types of manipulation performed by osteopaths and chiropractors or even some massage therapists may not be striking, depending on the practitioner and the patient being treated. A recent study lends some support to the use of "osteopathic" manipulation to treat low-back pain. Patients with low-back pain demonstrated that this kind of manipulation was equally effective when compared with standard medical care, such as muscle relaxants, analgesics, physical therapy, and TENS. Patients receiving osteopathic or standard medical treatment were quite pleased with their care and accepted their back problem well. However, those treated by standard care were more likely to spend more on medication and physical therapy, resulting in higher treatment costs. This study thus provides an economic argument for using spinal manipulation in treating certain kinds of low-back pain.

Osteopaths and chiropractors are trained differently. Chiropractors attend chiropractic colleges and receive degrees. They cannot prescribe medications or perform surgery and invasive procedures. Unlike chiropractors, osteopaths receive a degree (D.O., or Doctor of Osteopathy) that is the equivalent of a medical degree. They can and do prescribe medication and perform surgery and other invasive procedures, exactly as physicians with an M.D. degree. However, osteopaths also learn a form of spinal manipulation in their training that physicians with M.D.s do not learn.

Spending time and money on spinal manipulation or physical therapy twice a week for long periods of time usually may not be the best way to deal with chronic pain, especially if there are more definitive or less time-intensive therapies available. An effective medication regimen combined with a home exercise program is one alternative. In appropriate cases, decompressive surgery or other medical pain-relieving procedures, which may provide long-term benefits, should be considered as an alternative to years of chronic pain that does not respond well to anything else.

Even if spinal manipulation helps with low-back pain, I do think that people with head, neck, and shoulder pain should forgo manipulation of the neck for several reasons. Vigorous manipulation of the neck may damage the spinal cord of patients with spinal-cord compression from a disk, arthritic overgrowth, or a tumor. Spinal-cord damage can result in permanent neurological deficits, including paralysis. Manipulating an unstable spine can be disastrous, also damaging the fragile spinal cord within the bony spine. Chiropractors and massage therapists often do not obtain MRIs or other sophisticated radiological studies that would guide diagnosis and treatment. Chiropractors usually obtain simple X rays of the spine, but these may not always prevent them from manipulating an unstable spine. Plain X rays provide little information on conditions affecting the interior of the spine, such as stenosis, disk herniations, or tumors. Chiropractic manipulation of patients suffering from these problems provides little benefit and could be harmful.

Chiropractors have caused strokes by twisting the spine in such a way that arteries that pass through the bones of the upper spine to the brain become "kinked," thus closing off a vessel. Inadequate blood supply to the brain from a kinked vessel can result in a stroke, causing permanent neurological deficits, even in the young. A few years ago I treated a woman of twenty-seven who had suffered a stroke at the base of her brain, induced by chiropractic manipulation. She had risk factors for the stroke, including the fact that she was on the birth-control pill, smoked, had been taking certain decongestants, and had used cocaine shortly before the manipulation. She was under the care of a doctor who prescribed strong decongestants for chronic sinusitis, and she went to the chiropractor for control of her neck pain.

As soon as the chiropractor pulled her neck, she felt weakness and numbness in her face and part of one side of her body. Ultimately she recovered, returned to work, married, and had children. Only a patch of residual numbness in her face persisted. (As a sad commentary on our medical and legal systems, the chiropractor had no malpractice insurance to cover the cost of her medical bills, and her lawyer attempted to sue the physicians who initially treated her for the sinusitis and later for the stroke, because they were insured.)

KEY POINTS
About Nonmedical Pain Management

- Various low-risk, low-expense, and low-side-effect measures may provide pain relief, but in serious pain conditions relief may not be long-standing. Repeated treatments are often needed to provide ongoing relief.

- Certain types of treatment are not covered by some medical insurers. Medicare does not pay for acupuncture, for example.

- I do not advocate months of physical therapy, relaxation training, hypnosis, biofeedback, acupuncture, or spinal manipulation if these methods of treatment do not allow you to "graduate" to a healthier, less painful state of being, independent of ongoing treatment.

- The alternative/complementary treatments usually cannot hurt you, but that is no reason to undergo any treatment ineffective in relieving your pain.

- In mild to moderately painful conditions, if after two months these treatments are ineffective, seek some other form of therapy.

- For more severe pain that has not yet been treated by powerful medication or by surgery if needed, I recommend moving up the ladder more quickly rather than slowly.

3

Medication in the Treatment of Pain

Irrationally held truths may be more harmful than reasoned errors.

—THOMAS HENRY HUXLEY

Medication is useful only if physicians prescribe it appropriately and if you take it when needed. In the last century, and particularly in the last fifty years, there has been an explosive proliferation of highly effective, safe, well-tolerated pain-relieving medication. Sadly, in spite of these pharmacological advances, medication—narcotic and non-narcotic alike—is still all too often underprescribed by physicians and underutilized by patients.

After an operation, most patients are hooked up to intravenous medication (IV) with a patient-controlled analgesia (PCA) button they can push whenever they want medication—narcotics—for their acute postoperative pain. It is when these patients get out of the hospital that they will encounter prejudice about their pain if it becomes chronic. Regarding an elderly woman with ongoing pain following a successfully repaired hip fracture, an unaware orthopedist could say, "I fixed her hip six months ago. I don't know why she is in pain now. It must be psychological."

I maintain that her pain should be taken seriously and evaluated. If no apparent correctable cause can be found to relieve her symptoms, she should be treated with adequate pain medication for as long as necessary. This includes the long-term use of narcotics, if needed. In her case, part of the physician's role becomes one of controlling her pain so that she enjoys her remaining years fully. Prescribing medication like Percoset or similar substances on an ongoing basis is no different from giving medication to an asthmatic so he can walk around without wheezing.

Most doctors are reluctant to treat severe chronic pain with narcotics because they are afraid of government regulations about prescribing these drugs. They also have an exaggerated fear of addiction. Yet narcotics are the most effective medications for the treatment of most moderate to severe pain, and they are among the safest pain-relieving medications when taken appropriately. Their effectiveness may be greatly enhanced when combined with other pain medication, such as Tylenol (acetaminophen), and nonsteroidal medication, such as aspirin. Hopefully, with more enlightened education about pain and its treatment, including with narcotics, medical students (future generations of doctors), nurses, the public, and future government regulators will all understand that pain is a medical symptom in need of treatment. Just as elevated blood pressure or temperature would indicate treatment, so should pain.

For their part, patients are often as reluctant to use narcotics—the sinners' drugs—as some physicians are to prescribe these chemicals born of the opium dens. Most of my patients need encouragement to take as much medication as they need. Worse yet, I have seen patients who need and want to take narcotics but who are dissuaded by family members or friends afraid of addiction or of mental fogging. You can't imagine how many amateur doctors are lurking next door, each with an encyclopedia of misinformation.

Some people consider stoicism a virtue. They are reluctant to complain of pain, much less take any pain medication. If they complain of pain, they are afraid they will be considered "sissies" or weaklings. Men often think suffering in silence is "manly." Do you think Arnold Schwarzenegger wouldn't need narcotics if his leg broke due to a big tumor eating up the bone?

Others feel the medical staff won't like them if they complain.

To these patients who suffer under a misconception regarding narcotics, to the stoics who suffer in silence, and to those dreading disrespect from the medical staff, I tell you what I tell my patients. It is your job to complain and to consider treatments I propose, trying those that are most likely to both help and appeal to you. It is my task to attempt to treat your complaints with the best treatment medicine, anywhere in the world, can offer.

However, there are a few people who want medication to make them totally pain-free, and I have to educate them that they will have difficulty achieving this state without significant, intolerable side effects. For example, a condition like arthritis of the knee joints will get progressively worse. To survive with less pain, some patients will have to learn to accept less physical challenge, even on a good regimen of pain control. Dulling pain with medication is not always the whole answer to a complicated pain problem.

THE CHALLENGE OF FINDING THE DRUG THAT WORKS

Painkillers work either by diminishing conscious awareness of pain or by decreasing the formation or the transmission of pain impulses. Analogously, a car alarm continues to sound although we have closed the window and cannot hear it, or at least not as well. Medications that kill pain often are designed to mimic our body's own pain regulatory system (see chapter 1).

Pain management may involve treating the description of the disease rather than the disease. A throbbing headache indicates a vascular problem that should be treated with certain types of medication, from aspirin to sophisticated antimigraine medications. Burning or shocklike pain is often caused by irritated or damaged nerves and can be treated by anti-seizure medication and certain antidepressants. On the other hand, aching pain from muscular problems, a disk herniation, or a toothache is treated with anti-inflammatory drugs and, when severe, with narcotics.

Narcotics, certain antidepressants, and other drugs cause pain relief by inhibiting the function of specific pain-processing cells in the brain and spinal cord. These classes of drugs limit the number of pain messages that these cells can process, so you perceive less pain. The effect is similar to wearing earplugs in a noisy room. The more narcotics used, the less pain felt. For example, a surgeon can inflict excruciating damage to your body during an operation, but under anesthesia, the pain messages are either not delivered to the spinal cord or are not processed by the brain in a manner that prompts you to act on them.

When we begin to manage pain through medication, we must determine, sometimes through trial and error, the right drug or drugs and the correct dosage for a particular patient. We need to take into account his or her age and lifestyle and even, in some cases, figure out the best time and means of administering it. This process is an art, and there is more to it than what is taught in any book, including this one. While there are general principles, which this book is designed to present, each patient is unique. This is why it is so important for those in chronic pain to find a doctor who has successfully treated many patients with difficult-to-control pain.

I have had many patients who came to me with excruciating pain, taking pain medication that was ineffective yet caused unpleasant side effects. Some had left work and were considering going on permanent disability. A few felt that suicide might be the best way of getting out of their mess. In many cases, I was able to give them an effective pain regimen, including high doses of narcotics, anticonvulsants (medication designed originally to combat epilepsy), tricyclic antidepressants (used to control pain, not depression), and other medication. When needed, I had to treat considerable side effects, like constipation and sleepiness, with yet other drugs, so the patients could tolerate the beneficial effects of the pain medication. However, in most cases, I was able to put them back to work. Their treatment was complex but highly effective and quite tolerable.

Nonsteroidal Anti-inflammatory Drugs (NSAID)

Inflammation involves swelling, heat, redness, and pain. Nonsteroidal anti-inflammatory drugs (NSAIDs) reduce these symptoms in joints and soft tissues like the muscles, so at the right dosage they are effective in treating the pain of such conditions as arthritis, headache, and backache. Many are sold over the counter in dosages low enough not to require a prescription. The most common NSAID is aspirin. Don't confuse aspirin with Tylenol (acetaminophen), which is *not* an NSAID. Tylenol controls pain from arthritis and other conditions as well as the NSAIDs in many cases, but doesn't really have any anti-inflammatory properties. Tylenol will not damage the stomach, but can harm the liver in dosages above 4,000 mg a day. That would be almost thirteen 325-mg or eight 500-mg pills. Drinking considerable amounts of alcohol while consuming a lot of Tylenol on a chronic basis is a good way to end up searching for a liver transplant.

The NSAID ibuprofen is the generic form of Advil or Motrin, which often helps with the pain of menstruation, among other complaints. Another NSAID, naproxen, is available as Aleve. At any dose, all these NSAID drugs interfere with the ability of the blood to clot. (Stop taking them ten days before surgery or invasive procedures to restore your normal blood-clotting mechanism.) At high doses, or with prolonged use, particularly in women over sixty-five, NSAIDs can cause nausea, indigestion, and ulcer formation. They can also cause liver and kidney damage and mild water retention—enough to put some patients with frail hearts into heart failure, a condition in which water accumulates in their lungs.

These drugs are the most widely used pain relievers and many in this class, like the ones mentioned above, may even be bought without a prescription. Yet they probably account for more deaths every year than prescribed narcotics, which are erroneously thought to be the really dangerous drugs. There are at least 16,500 deaths each year in the United States and Canada in the population of arthritis patients taking NSAIDs. (Obviously, people who are not arthritis patients also take these drugs.) This figure represents as many deaths annually as those due to asthma, cervical cancer, and melanoma combined, and one-third as many deaths annually as those due to AIDS. In the same countries, there are also 107,000 annual hospitalizations due to severe gastrointestinal side effects from NSAID use. (The COX-2 inhibitors discussed below could significantly reduce these horrible statistics.)

NSAIDs relieve pain by blocking production of the enzyme cyclooxygenase (COX), which helps produce irritating prostaglandins as part of the inflammatory process. The COX enzyme has two forms. Blocking either COX-1 or COX-2 reduces pain. However, COX-1 has a protective effect on the stomach lining. Blocking this enzyme removes this protector, allowing ulcers to form. That is why most NSAIDs have sometimes had serious gastrointestinal side effects, including bleeding. COX-2 can be blocked without as much risk of gastrointestinal side effects and with the same level of pain relief obtained by blocking COX-1.

COX-2 inhibitor drugs are a new class of NSAIDs that block only COX-2 without affecting COX-1. As painkillers, they are only as effective as regular NSAIDs (nonselective COX-1 and COX-2 inhibitors). They are more expensive and should be used on patients who have ulcers or indigestion or are likely to develop these conditions with other NSAIDs. If COX-2 inhibitors (drugs with brand names such as Celebrex and Vioxx) live up to their promise, patients with ulcers, gastritis, and esophagitis as well as elderly women will be able to take an NSAID without hurting their gastrointestinal system.

Corticosteroids

Corticosteroids are man-made drugs that are chemically similar to active hormones produced by the adrenal glands. Because they reduce inflammation and swelling, they control musculoskeletal pain from joints, pain from compressed nerves (such as "sciatica"), and pain from bones invaded by cancerous metastasized tumors. They are far more powerful than NSAIDs, and so are their side effects.

In pain control, corticosteroids are used only for a brief period of a few weeks because they stress the gastrointestinal tract and because of their serious long-term side effects. However, they are sometimes used for longer periods to treat certain kinds of arthritis, some conditions in which the body attacks itself, cancer-related bone or nerve pain, and tumors involving the brain or spinal cord (see chapter 10).

Side effects of taking corticosteroids for more than a few weeks are increased appetite and weight gain, ulcers, and insomnia. Women on oral steroids can experience menstrual irregularities. As time passes, the side effects include water retention with swelling of the legs, acne, increased risk of infections due to diminished immunity, and steroid-related diabetes. Some patients on steroids develop psychiatric disturbances, including mania and depression.

Osteoporosis, weakness of the muscles (particularly in the thighs), breakdown of the skin, and changes in distribution of body fat, such as lumps of fat appearing on the back, are other side effects. Most of these are reversible once the steroids are discontinued. However, destruction of the hip joints may occur with long-term steroid use, requiring joint replacement. Obviously, all these side effects compromise the body to varying degrees, so the less time you can be on corticosteroids the better.

These steroids can be taken orally, but they are often injected. This causes the medication to remain concentrated in one area for a while, such as the inside of the spine (epidurals, placed into the fat-containing space within the spine, around the spinal cord and nerves) and joints (knees, hips, or shoulders). Eventually the medicine leaks back into the body, of course, and its local effect dissipates. Steroid treatment reduces the inflammation for a short period, during which time a condition can heal, but for an ongoing process like arthritis, the condition continues and the pain often returns.

Tricyclic Antidepressants

Tricyclics were originally used only to treat depression but later were found to work on several chemical pathways of the central nervous system, reducing the input of pain messages to the brain. They increase the level of two naturally occurring substances—serotonin and norepinephrine—in the brain and spinal cord. These substances inhibit neurons in the spinal cord that transmit pain signals up to the brain so fewer pain impulses are processed by the brain.

Pain can be treated with a far lower dose of these tricyclics than is prescribed for psychiatric reasons. Also, the pain-relieving effects become apparent within five days, while their antidepressant effect, at higher doses, may not begin for several weeks. It would appear that they work differently on different parts of the central nervous system in alleviating pain as opposed to depression.

Trycyclics such as Elavil (amitriptyline), Pamelor (nortriptyline), Tofranil (imipramine), and Norpramin (desipramine) work on pain from nerve damage due to:

- diabetes, AIDS, and strokes

- cancer and chemotherapy

- spinal cord injury, shingles, neuromas, and scarred nerves

- damage to a nerve root caused by disk herniation or surgical trauma

As well as forms of musculoskeletal pain such as:

- temporomandibular joint dysfunction (TMJ)

- fibromyalgia

Tricyclics are easy to take. Once the proper dosage is found, it does not change over time and one pill once or twice a day is enough. They can be combined easily with other pain-relieving medication as needed.

Best of all, many people can tolerate at least one of the tricyclics well. They vary in side effects, with Elavil being the most sedating and most likely to cause other side effects, such as dry mouth and blood-pressure problems. Norpramin usually has fewer side effects, but it may be more likely to cause insomnia, disturbingly vivid dreams, and some degree of agitation. I prefer to prescribe Pamelor for most patients and rarely use Elavil, because of the significant sedation and other side effects associated with it.

All tricyclics may cause dry mouth; Elavil is the most and Norpramin the least likely to cause this, with Pamelor in the middle. The same drugs similarly cause blood pressure changes, following the pattern of dry mouth. They can cause some people—usually the elderly—to feel faint when standing up, as when getting out of bed. They all may cause weight gain, which over time can become a problem. Rarely, women may develop menstrual irregularities and even begin to produce milk, and men may develop sexual dysfunction. As a rule, these drugs should not be used if you have heart-rhythm disturbance, glaucoma, or an enlarged prostate.

Some of the side effects of the tricyclics may be exploited for therapeutic purposes. The more sedating Elavil may be useful in reducing agitation due to pain or other problems and also may promote nighttime sleep, which is not always a bad thing for patients with severe pain.

The Newest Antidepressants: Prozac and Her Daughters

There's a whole new group of antidepressants called selective serotonin receptor inhibitors (SSRIs), made famous by Prozac (fluoxetine). Members of this family are used for all sorts of things—depression, shyness, panic attacks. Everyone reading this book knows someone taking a drug in this family, which includes Prozac, Paxil (paroxetine), Effexor (venlaxafine), Zoloft (sertraline), and Welbutrin (bupropion).

They appear overall to be less effective than tricyclic antidepressants in treating pain. They do have fewer major side effects than the older tricyclic-type antidepressants, but they may have annoying side effects such as weight gain, minor sleep disturbance, and inability to attain orgasm or ejaculate.

Obviously, the catch here is that not all antidepressants have good pain-relieving qualities. However, relieving depression and anxiety, both common symptoms associated with chronic pain, also helps to relieve the physical pain. If these drugs help depression better than a tricyclic, or are better tolerated, by all means they should be used, possibly in combination with low doses of a tricyclic in some cases. By lessening the depression associated with chronic pain, you may feel better overall. We need some research to come up with drugs that are effective and safe in treating both pain and depression simultaneously.

Anticonvulsants or Antiseizure Drugs

Neuropathic pain (see chapter 7), such as severe, jabbing, electrical pain in the face from trigeminal neuralgia, can be treated with drugs called anticonvulsants or antiseizure medicines. A seizure is an "explosion" of overactive brain cells. Neuropathic pain usually involves one or several overactive or overly excitable nerves—peripheral nerves, nerves in the central nervous system, or both. Anticonvulsants stop abnormal firing of overactive nerves. The nervous system transmits information electro-chemically, and neuropathic pain is like a seizure in certain nerves brought on by a short circuit or "sparking" in wires of a sensitized nervous system.

Phenytoin (Dilantin), carbamazepine (Tegretol), gabapentin (Neu-rontin), and valproic acid (Depakote) are four popularly used anti-seizure medications that treat the pain of irritable or damaged nerves by reducing the "sparking." However, not everyone, particularly the elderly, can tolerate dosages high enough to treat neuropathic pain.

This is particularly unfortunate because many forms of neuropathic pain affect the elderly, such as diabetic neuropathy, postherpetic neu-ralgia (following shingles), or trigeminal neuralgia (a form of facial neuropathic pain). Many elderly patients taking Tegretol have queasi-ness and walk as if they were drunk, even on a low dose. I try to avoid giving Tegretol to older patients except those with trigeminal neural-gia, in which case Tegretol is the most effective drug. Instead I give them Neurontin, even though they have to take it four times a day and it takes longer to find a pain-relieving dosage than with Tegretol. The most common side effect from Neurontin is sleepiness, and when that side effect becomes bothersome, I do not raise the dosage or I raise it very slowly. Taking Neurontin as well as a tricyclic antidepressant can be helpful, if either drug alone is insufficiently effective.

If that doesn't work, I may add Tegretol to Neurontin and a tri-cyclic. Many patients, particularly the elderly, don't like taking all these pills on top of the other medication they may be taking, includ-ing cardiac and blood-pressure medication and drugs for osteoporosis, hiatal hernia, diabetes, and so on. Some of the drugs, like Neurontin, are quite expensive, a particularly thorny issue for the elderly, who are often on low fixed incomes.

Certain of the anticonvulsants, and some other drugs useful for treating neuropathic pain, work by manipulating a neurotransmitter called GABA, which inhibits the transmission of pain impulses in the central nervous system. When it binds to receptors on a cell, the cell is inhibited from firing. It inhibits the firing of second neurons in the pain pathway, which would normally carry pain impulses from the spinal cord up to the brain (see chapter 1).

Valium-like drugs such as Klonopin (clonazepam), used for panic attacks and seizure control, appear to enhance the activity of GABA. Putting it simply, GABA becomes more potent in the presence of molecules of Klonopin. The anticonvulsants Depakote and Neurontin both increase brain GABA levels. Lioresal (baclofen), a drug used to treat spastic or tight muscles caused by brain or spinal-cord damage (as seen in cerebral palsy or multiple sclerosis), acts like GABA. Klonopin, the two anticonvulsants mentioned above, and baclofen have been used with some success in controlling neuropathic pain.

Antiarrhythmics or Sodium Channel Blockers

Certain sodium channel blockers control abnormal rhythms of the heart. The heart functions electrically like the nervous system. These blockers, such as Mexitil (mexiletine) and Tonocard (tocainide), not only control abnormal electrical activity in the heart, but can stop the abnormal painful firing of damaged nerves and control transmission of pain impulses. I have had two patients with trigeminal neuralgia whose disease was controlled with Tegretol for a long time. When this drug no longer worked, they responded to nothing else but Mexitil. These drugs are not without potential cardiac side effects and they can damage the liver. They should not be used until other drugs such as tricyclics and anticonvulsants have failed. However, they can usually be used in very low doses effectively and safely, alone or in combination with other pain medication, in the treatment of neuropathic pain.

Ultram

A relatively new drug called tramadol (Ultram) is a painkiller that binds to opioid receptors in the nervous system, mimicking a narcotic, and also manipulates norepinephrine and serotonin, like the tricyclic antidepressants. In spite of its dual action, it is only about as powerful as codeine, used for mild to moderate pain, such as that seen after some dental procedures. It may help control various types of pain, ranging from musculoskeletal to nerve related (neuropathic). However, the concept behind this drug—working on more than one pain-controlling system at the same time—is intriguing and may be exploited to better advantage with other drugs in the future.

Ultram is not a narcotic, but because it binds to the opioid receptors in the brain, it may cause addiction in those predisposed to this problem. It causes sleepiness and constipation, too, for the same reason.

Dextromethorphan

Dextromethorphan is an active ingredient in some cough syrups. It suppresses coughs. But it also blocks a type of receptor—which we will call the "excitatory receptor," a villain in the drama of pain, especially neuropathic pain. These excitatory receptors are stimulated by certain excitatory neurotransmitters—aspartate and glutamate. These neurotransmitters begin pain transmission in the spinal cord when they are released by the axon terminals of peripheral nerves, exciting the second neurons in the pain pathway. The second neurons, in turn, cause pain impulses to go up to the brain along their long axons.

Dextromethorphan may nip this process in the bud by blocking the excitatory receptor and thereby blocking pain transmission. Its effects are not spectacular in the clinical setting, because of the drug's side effects. In the doses needed to diminish neuropathic pain, this drug causes unacceptable drowsiness. However, it opens a window of opportunity to develop safe, effective excitatory-receptor-blocking drugs.

Pain-Relieving Skin Creams

Certain injectable local anesthetics are now being applied to the skin in creams and medication-soaked patches (like a nicotine patch). Emla cream contains lidocaine and prilocaine, two local anesthetics. A new product called Lidoderm is a patch containing lidocaine. The patches and creams soaked with local anesthetic have been used to help control the pain of postherpetic neuralgia and various procedures involving the skin, such as insertion of intravenous catheters in a scared child.

Capsaicin, a derivative from chili peppers, has been put into Zostrix, a pain-relieving cream. The drug in this cream doesn't mimic a molecule at a receptor or stimulate the release or action of a molecule at the axon terminal. Instead, capsaicin may control pain in a way not previously seen in this chapter—depleting another pain-inducing excitatory neurotransmitter called Substance P. It exists both in the receptor end of the peripheral nerve as well as its axon tip within the spinal cord.

The major effect of capsaicin is at the peripheral nerve endings (figure 1). In the periphery, Substance P is released in response to injury. It stimulates the peripheral nerve ending to fire transmitting pain impulses up the nerve to the spinal cord. It also causes inflammatory changes in the skin and underlying tissues, and local swelling and redness by making small blood vessels dilate and leak. It may even be partially responsible for both the pain and soft tissue changes that occur in diseases like rheumatoid arthritis. Capsaicin excites chemical receptors in the skin on which it is rubbed. Remember, it is derived from chili peppers and feels a bit like peppers in the skin. Peripheral Substance P is activated by the drug, stimulating receptors to transmit pain impulses up the peripheral nerve to the axon terminal, inducing it to fire. Substance P is also released into the spinal cord, exciting the second neurons in the pain pathway, which transmit the burning sensation to the brain. This process continues for several weeks, during which the cream is applied several times daily. The patient experiences continual peppery burning, on top of the original pain—from diabetic neuropathy, for example. Eventually, less pain is felt from both the underlying neuropathy and the pepper cream. How does this occur?

The pepper cream, by "overworking" the Substance P system, wears it out, depleting the neurotransmitter. By reducing the amount of Substance P, especially at the peripheral nerve endings, less Substance P is available to cause pain transmission. Substance P causes local swelling by making blood vessels expand and leak. Capsaicin also depletes this peripheral Substance P.

This cream is also used in postherpetic neuralgia (see chapter 7) and may help alleviate what is called pathological itching—the annoying problem of areas that itch for no reason. Zostrix may alleviate pain in various painful neuropathies, sometimes with good effect. It may be tried on the painful joints of rheumatoid and osteoarthritis. Don't get it in your eyes. You will feel they went to hell for a brief period, although it shouldn't damage them. In the future, a more effective means of depleting or inhibiting Substance P may be developed, replacing this cumbersome cream.

TREATING PAIN WITH NARCOTICS

Imagine that you have found the perfect, life-enhancing gift to give a friend, but it must be wrapped in three sheets of paper. Before your friend can reach the gift, he must examine each paper and read its message. The first sheet of wrapping tells him that refusing gifts is a sign of strong and admirable character and that he must refuse gifts if he wants to be a "real man." The second says that the contents of your gift will cause him to become a drug addict, which could lead to various forms of degradation and at best a period of painful, horrific withdrawal. The third wrapping, if he has gotten this far without running away, informs him that the gift is so dangerous that it must be regulated by the government. In fact, a government representative may be preparing to investigate him even as he reads.

This story pretty much represents the position of many patients in significant chronic pain. Helping someone find and accept the proper narcotic drugs for debilitating chronic pain is mixed up with ideas of personal weakness, images of addiction and its associated lifestyle, and government regulation.

How Narcotics Work

Narcotics work and have side effects for the same reason. In the early 1970s, two medical scientists at Johns Hopkins, Drs. Solomon Snyder and Candice Pert, discovered receptors for narcotics or opioids in the brains of mice. A bit later, another group of scientists discovered certain protein molecules called endorphins, which fit like a key into a lock, the lock being the receptors. The relationship between these endorphins and our own pain control was thus demonstrated. However, opioid receptors were found in other organs as well, and it was surmised that these receptors play a role in all sorts of bodily functions, including pain, pleasure, and the degree of dependence on and tolerance to opiates.

Narcotics like morphine are not perfect three-dimensional molecular matches for our own opioids. They are keys, which fit the lock imperfectly. Yes, they fit well enough to provide great pain relief, but they also fit into other locks or receptors that have nothing to do with pain control, and that is the basis for their side effects. It is the binding to receptors in the base of the brain, which influence the gastrointestinal tract, that cause some people to have nausea, at least transiently, and almost all patients to have constipation when taking narcotics. Similarly, receptors to which man-made narcotics bind may depress respiration, another potential side effect. Some narcotics may alter your mood by binding to still other receptors.

Not all narcotics bind to receptors in the same way in each person. Some patients may tolerate morphine, Dilaudid (hydromorphinone), and fentanyl (used in Duragesic skin patches), three different narcotics, without a significant problem. In other cases, a patient may tolerate morphine but vomit when taking Dilaudid or fentanyl. Incidentally, the latter drug appears to cause 30 percent less nausea and constipation than other narcotics—it bonds to certain receptors less than its narcotic colleagues.

A crucial issue with narcotic drugs is tolerance. Tolerance means a drug's effect decreases over time, presumably because of some physical change—a reduction in the number of receptors for a drug or a change in the configuration of the receptor, the lock for the drug's molecular key.

The good news is that most people become tolerant of many side effects of narcotic drugs within one or two weeks (except constipation,

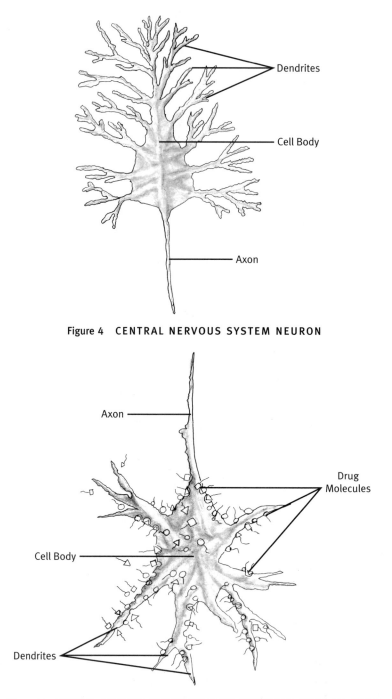

Figure 4 CENTRAL NERVOUS SYSTEM NEURON

Figure 5 CENTRAL NERVOUS SYSTEM NEURON SHOWING SIMILAR DRUG
MOLECULES BINDING TO DIFFERENT TYPES OF RECEPTORS

which usually has to be treated on a long-term basis) while still obtaining good pain relief. The reason for this differential tolerance is not clear. Perhaps the interaction of many narcotics with the receptors causing side effects is different from the interaction with the receptors causing pain relief.

The bad news is that some patients also become tolerant to the pain-relieving properties of a narcotic. If this occurs, changing to another narcotic that binds to our pain-relieving narcotic receptors differently may help better control the pain. This strategy may fool or outwit the mechanism of tolerance.

Man-made narcotics are more potent than our own natural opioids, the endorphins, but both work along the same lines. If you were taking morphine when you touched a hot stove, your reaction to the heat would be slower than if you didn't take the pain reliever. It may take more heat to make you jump and you might jump away more slowly. You still would jump, however, and learn not to touch the hot stove in the future. Once you have been treated with morphine, the pain-transmitting cells in the spinal cord are forced to slow down. They are inhibited from rapidly firing in response to the incoming barrage of pain signals, which are carried into the spinal cord along the nerve coming from your burned finger. The morphine acts like a brake, modulating or inhibiting an important segment of the pain-transmission system.

Why Most People Won't Become Addicted to Narcotic Pain Treatment

Remember that first cigarette behind the garage? Boy, did it make you green. Your body wasn't used to it. If you were foolish enough to keep smoking, you got used to the effect of nicotine—tolerant to it. You wouldn't feel green, and would want to smoke more cigarettes, and even feel terrible if you didn't have any. You became dependent on nicotine. Worse yet, you might have grown to crave them, purely because you liked to smoke or liked the way smoking made you feel. That craving is addiction, often confused with tolerance and dependence.

Tolerance means that the body adapts to an opiate so that both therapeutic and side effects are diminished. Fortunately, tolerance to the side effects of opiates develops relatively quickly but tolerance to the pain-relieving effects of these drugs develops slowly, for unclear reasons. Most chronic pain, once controlled, may be treated with a stable dose that never has to be increased. In practical terms, someone in chronic pain may take the equivalent of six to eight Percosets daily for years, with good results and few side effects. He gets used to the drug.

If a person not used to that amount of narcotic took it, he would be sleepy and act as if overdosed.

Dependence is physical adaptation to the presence of a drug, narcotic or non-narcotic. Has someone in your office ever decided to go off caffeine for a while? Why, a person can become a bear—jittery and headachy. You've seen them. If coffee drinkers go without their drug, they will have some withdrawal symptoms—just like withdrawal from narcotics.

Dependence and tolerance are normal physiological adaptations to the exposure of the central nervous system and the rest of the body to a chemical on a regular basis. Now, the real bugaboo with narcotics is *addiction*. What does it make you think of? Dazed people lying around an opium den or in a filthy crack house? Drugs are not paving the road to hell when they are prescribed for the medical control of pain. Addiction, by any definition, is compulsive, inappropriate use of a drug *for a psychological reason*—to get high. Use for pain control is not addiction.

The most commonly abused drugs in the United States that result in emergency-room visits for overdose are cocaine, heroin, and Valium-like drugs, in that order. Notice the conspicuous absence of any prescription narcotics from the top of the list.

Pseudo-addiction is drug-seeking behavior by patients whose pain is not adequately controlled. The nurse complains, "That kid down in room 404 who keeps asking for her pain medication must be an addict." No, she was just in a bad motorcycle accident and broke a leg, which needed open surgery to repair, and skinned half the upper layer of flesh off her back. Her doctor prescribed oral narcotics every six hours as needed, in spite of the fact that the medication only lasts three to four hours. He also prescribed about half the amount of narcotic she needs to take the edge off, much less make her truly comfortable. That kid in 404 may be obnoxious outside the hospital for other reasons, but now she is whining because she is in excruciating pain and cannot imagine how she'll ever get comfortable, much less go to sleep. Most patients in pain asking for more narcotics are undermedicated. Don't ever forget that. Her demand for more drugs is pseudo-addiction. Real addiction is when a person demands a drug whether or not she is in pain.

In a study of national databases, the use and abuse of five narcotics, including fentanyl, Dilaudid, Demerol (meperidine), morphine, and oxycodone, the narcotic in Percoset, were studied from 1990 to 1996. Use of these drugs increased severalfold while abuse decreased. The trend clearly demonstrates increasing medical use of narcotics for pain control and no associated increase in narcotic abuse. The trend obviously should continue.

Why Your Physician Won't Prescribe Narcotics

Vastly exaggerated fear of addiction is one major reason physicians underprescribe narcotics. An even more important impediment to the medical use of narcotics is a very real physician concern regarding bureaucratic audits and punitive government regulations. In thirty-one states, doctors can be prosecuted by state and local law-enforcement agencies for *over*prescribing narcotics to treat pain. The definition of overprescribing is often without basis in terms of contemporary professional understanding of pain management. Understandably, too many physicians are unwilling to prescribe narcotics, avoiding the costly office record keeping required for writing these prescriptions, not to mention the exceedingly expensive potential of defending themselves in a bureaucratic audit or legal investigation. Tragically for patients, many physicians are more likely to capitulate to their fear of punitive regulatory oversight, prescribing ineffective, non-narcotic medication. Interestingly, since 1997, twenty-five states have enacted laws to protect physicians and their patients. Unfortunately, the other states haven't.

Fear of addiction should not prevent you from getting pain relief. In a survey conducted for the American Academy of Pain Medicine and the American Pain Society, published in 1999, 49 percent of those who had taken narcotic pain relievers said they were concerned about addiction. The vast majority of patients with pain from cancer or other causes do not become addicted to narcotics they take chronically for that pain (fewer than 5 percent become addicted, according to some data).

You, the public, must work to foster the commonplace, appropriate use of prescribed narcotics to treat pain, especially chronic pain. Within your communities, strive to alter *irrational* beliefs concerning addiction to prescribed narcotics. Prod the larger political system to liberalize regulations controlling the medical use of narcotics.

Balancing Pain Relief and Side Effects

In evaluating what kinds of side effects are acceptable, you have to weigh what is wrong with you, what medications and procedures can help your prognosis, what the chances are that your condition will improve on its own, and whether your pain is chronic.

Severe nausea and vomiting are not acceptable side effects of narcotics, but a little queasiness for a few days is. Most patients get used to most narcotic side effects in one week, except for constipation, which will not go away but can be treated. It is not acceptable to be drowsy or so sedated that you walk like a drunk. If you are on a new drug regimen and sleepy for a few hours of the day, but for the first time in years you have 75 percent reduction of chronic, severe, otherwise intractable pain, then the pain relief outweighs the side effects. That's how doctors weigh side effects. It's common sense.

Side effects from narcotics may be treated and often disappear with time because of tolerance. Nausea may be treated with antinausea medications like Compazine (prochlorperazine) and sleepiness may be counteracted on a long-term basis with amphetamines. Constipation is usually a persistent problem that may be controlled with a high-fiber diet, lots of fluids, a stool softener, and possibly a laxative.

The most serious side effect of narcotics—slowing of respiration and buildup of deadly carbon dioxide from inadequate breathing—is quite rare if narcotics are used as prescribed. Obviously if someone wants to commit suicide by taking all of their Percoset at once, they could die, or end up with brain damage from severe narcotic-induced depression of respiratory function.

Take the dose of the drug you need to control your pain. You should be given a drug that controls your pain with minimal long-term side effects. Realize that you can have side effects with one member of a drug family and none with another drug in that same group. Narcotics like Dilaudid, Percoset, methadone, codeine, and fentanyl skin patches (Duragesic) all may substitute for morphine and for one another. If one drug doesn't work or isn't tolerated, try another.

How to Use Narcotics Effectively

Preparations of morphine last from three to four hours, eight to twelve hours, or twenty-four hours. On the other hand, fentanyl patches (Duragesic) last three days.

The strength of a drug, in relation to how it is given, depends on the amount of drug that gets to the pain-modulating areas of the spinal cord and brain. When a drug like morphine is given by mouth, it is absorbed by the small intestine and goes to the liver, where it is broken down before circulating to the brain and spinal cord. When given intravenously, more drug gets into the brain and spinal cord before it is broken down, so a lower dose will provide the same pain relief as a larger dose given by mouth. Intraspinal injection of morphine permits still less of the drug to be given with good pain relief, because the drug is delivered close to its site of action—the cells with opioid receptors in the spinal cord that modulate or inhibit pain transmission.

In many difficult-to-control pain states, drugs can be used in combination. You may need a long-acting narcotic and a short-acting one, plus some other drug to work more specifically on neuropathic pain and one or several drugs to control the side effects of the narcotics (most commonly constipation).

In many cases of musculoskeletal pain—like a chronically painful back—a narcotic can be combined with nonsteroidal drugs like acetaminophen (Tylenol) to achieve better pain relief with less narcotic and fewer narcotic side effects. Narcotics and NSAIDs act on different pain-relieving mechanisms. As it turns out, adding an NSAID to a narcotic has a synergistic effect, which is more than an additive effect.

Prozac and similar antidepressants can accelerate the metabolism or breakdown of narcotics. Patients using these may require more narcotics, not because they are depressed drug addicts, but because their narcotics don't last as long.

Physicians must know not only the duration of pain-relieving activity of various drugs but also their strength. Just as Scotch is stronger than sherry, and pure grain alcohol stronger than Scotch, Percoset is twice as strong as morphine, and Dilaudid six to seven times stronger than morphine. If, despite experiencing relief, a patient doesn't tolerate 60 mg of morphine because of side effects or even a skin reaction to the drug, 30 mg of Percoset may be substituted.

Timing medicine correctly is as important as finding the correct medication. If you know a pill takes forty-five minutes to work, don't wait until your back hurts to take it. Anticipate what you are going to do and take your medicine before you take a walk or play with little children or go shopping, so that the medicine will be in effect when the pain starts. This will also keep your dosage down. If a medication works for about four hours, watch the clock. Be aware that around four hours after the dose you should take it again before the first pill wears off. Otherwise, you are going to have pain in the middle of your Christmas-shopping spree and you will squirm until your pill takes effect.

Even here, however, there is room for an exception. Some people who are heavily medicated for chronic pain say it does slow down their thinking. They deliberately take short-acting drugs that they allow to wear off in order to give them periods when their thinking is sharper, despite the pain they experience. Except for these rare cases, I urge my patients to avoid the seesaw of taking medicine, eventually obtaining pain relief, and having it wear off, experiencing new pain, and so forth.

Relief of chronic pain can take time and it involves communication and trust between doctor and patient, as well as patience. For example, of the drugs I have mentioned, it may take two months to figure out the proper dosage of Neurontin, because if the dose is raised too quickly, severe sleepiness may occur. It can take at least two weeks to experience the pain-relieving effects of anticonvulsants like Dilantin and Tegretol. Reaching the proper dose of tricyclics like Pamelor may take one to three weeks. That is a relatively short period, but not for a person suffering through side effects and waiting for pain relief.

METHODS OF DELIVERY

Narcotics may be delivered in the form of pills, liquids, or candies; nasal sprays; rectal suppositories; skin patches; subcutaneously, or under the skin; intramuscularly; intravenously; and into the spine. For any given narcotic, the more drug that reaches the brain and spinal cord quickly, the greater and quicker the pain relief. When you take a narcotic by mouth, it requires about forty-five minutes to be absorbed and digested. Some of the drug is even destroyed by the digestive process, so less of it is available to diminish pain. Narcotics introduced directly into the bloodstream do not have to be digested like a pill, so more medication is delivered quickly. In fact, narcotics administered by the subcutaneous or intravenous route are three to six times more potent than the same dose given by mouth. Morphine injected into the epidural space (the fatty layer within the spine) is about ten times more effective as that given intravenously. However, the same drug delivered into the fluid bathing the brain and spinal cord, is *one hundred* times more potent than it is when given intravenously.

Skin Patches. The Duragesic skin patch is a user-friendly means of delivering medication. The patch takes about twelve to eighteen hours to kick in and about the same time to wear off if you decide to remove it. The medication in each patch lasts about three days in most patients and as little as two days in some. Fentanyl, the potent narcotic in these patches, is several hundred times stronger than morphine, yet fentanyl causes 30 percent less nausea and constipation than other narcotics. This patch has liberated many patients, especially those with cancer, from the inconvenience of intravenous morphine and, in some cases, more high-tech means of intraspinal pain control—even in the hospital.

The following invasive methods of drug delivery should be used **when pain can't be controlled otherwise in a tolerable fashion.**

Subcutaneous Delivery. This route involves delivering narcotics into the fat under the skin with a needle. Chronically administered medication is delivered by a small, portable pump connected through thin tubing to the implanted needle. It is easier to maintain and less expensive than the IV route, lending itself to outpatient and hospice use.

Intravenous Delivery. Cancer pain in a hospital setting or pain following surgery is often managed with intravenous narcotics. Patients often manage their own narcotic infusions with patient-controlled analgesia (PCA). Using a small push-button device, you control the amount of narcotic you use, within a prescribed range, depending on your minute-to-minute needs. Intravenous systems can be used at home as well.

Intraspinal Delivery. Less drug can be given with better pain control and fewer side effects using the intraspinal route. There is a tremendous benefit in the use of intraspinal narcotics in the right patient, such as one who has received a high dose of medication, by less invasive methods, that is ineffective or poorly tolerated. For some, intraspinal pain-relieving medication is a lifesaver. (Remember, pain may not kill you, but it may make you wish you were dead.)

To administer intraspinal medication, a catheter must be implanted into the epidural space or the spinal fluid through which pain-relieving medication may be injected at regular intervals. This is how anesthesiologists give intraspinal medication for surgery or during childbirth. For patients requiring chronic intraspinal medication, a pump can be implanted into the body to deliver the drugs continuously. These implanted pump systems are somewhat technically difficult to maintain, but they can achieve good results. Once such a device has been implanted, you are married to it—and to the physician who maintains it. Beware of any physician who seems too eager to use this technology early in your saga of chronic pain instead of moderate to high doses of effective, well-tolerated oral narcotics or skin patches. You can get divorced from the device, but it's a bit of a task.

A Soldier's Story

I treated a retired Israeli soldier for severe back and leg pain due to arachnoiditis—scarring of the covering of the nerves in the lumbar spine. It resulted from a bad reaction to an old myelogram, carried out with a now obsolete X-ray dye. He had come to me for a spinal-cord stimulator (see chapter 10), which he didn't really want and perhaps didn't need. I tried to treat him with various narcotics and other non-narcotic drugs, initially with good effect. Then he developed an allergic rash and felt nauseated. He also had no appetite. I eliminated most drugs and switched the remaining narcotics to some sister drugs. Still he developed a rash and had a host of other miserable side effects. I had tried morphine and oxycodone (the narcotic in Percoset), and both caused an allergic response.

Then I tried a different type of narcotic—the Duragesic skin patch. It was supposed to be used every three days. Lo and behold, it worked like a charm. He felt significant pain relief and I breathed easier. He called me two weeks later from Israel to inform me that the drug seemed to last only two and a half days, not the three as prescribed. Did I call him an addict or accuse him of trying to get more drugs? No. I not only believed him but told him the truth—a small percentage of patients may need to change their patch every two and a half or even, in some cases, every two days.

So, now he changes his patch every two days and appears to be doing well. In the meantime, we've been able to start him gingerly on a second drug, Neurontin, trying to further help him. We are both quite pleased with his progress. I am pleased that he recognized the potential to be helped with medication and had the patience and confidence in me to stick it out during the trial-and-error period.

Around-the-Clock Narcotics for Chronic Pain

For the many who require chronic medication with a fairly high dose of narcotics, there are long-acting forms of narcotics that last eight to twelve hours, as well as patches that last three days. This allows a patient to have a continuing level of painkilling narcotic in his blood—and at the site of action in the brain and spinal cord—for a longer period of time. This gives the pain receptors continued exposure to narcotics. For an unbearable spurt of pain, a shorter-acting drug can be added.

Most important, you require less drug in twenty-four hours if you allow the blood level—and ultimately brain concentration—of the drug to remain in a therapeutic range. However sensible this may be, some people resist. A little more than one-fifth of patients with severe to chronic pain said they do not take their medications as prescribed because they want to control the amount or because they want to take them only when they are "needed."

What severe pain sufferers need is around-the-clock medication.

Many should judiciously combine shorter- and longer-acting narcotics to keep their blood level within a certain range, which minimizes "breakthrough pain"—an explosion of pain not controlled by the long-acting drugs. If someone needs a drug every three hours, he is misguided to wait six hours to take it. As we have seen, patients can understandably become very irritable—nearly unmanageable by cold institutional guidelines of decorum and efficiency—until their pain is controlled.

The goal of pain management is to end discomfort so patients can keep working productively and enjoy their family, friends, and personal interests. If patients can live on a regimen of properly prescribed narcotics for the rest of their lives, and this enables them to enjoy their spouse or loved ones fully, pick up their children, drive a car, work in a full capacity, and play a sport, they should do so.

Sadly, the strongest treatments most patients in severe pain get is all-purpose headache medication like Tylenol, nonsteroidals like ibuprofen, or weak, less regulated narcotics like codeine. In fact, on average, it takes most Americans in moderate to severe chronic pain one and a half years to get relief from their pain. What do you think the most effective drugs are to solve this problem? Right, narcotics. Why does it take so long to get relief? Because too many members of my profession and society at large won't deal with the N word.

MEDICATION AND AGING

Flexibility in manipulating various pain medications is important in dealing with younger patients. It is an absolute necessity in treating the elderly or any patients with serious illnesses affecting multiple bodily systems. The American Geriatric Society advocates both long- and short-acting narcotics for the treatment of moderate to severe pain. Yet it is estimated that 50 to 90 percent of the elderly live with unrelieved pain.

Medication has done wonders to alleviate painful conditions, but as the body ages, it tolerates drugs less well and is more susceptible to side effects like sleepiness, nausea, and constipation. Elderly people are likely to have more than one medical condition. A doctor has to be careful about giving them medication that could cause them to be drowsy, increasing the danger of falling and breaking a hip or developing a blood clot over the brain. People with severe emphysema—many of whom are elderly—who take the narcotics *improperly,* may become sleepy and confused. They could even die, although this should not occur from *properly* prescribed narcotics.

The role of physicians is to find the right drug or other treatment for a patient's pain, regardless of the difficulty age or medical conditions may impose.

A Nurse's Story

A delightful young nurse practitioner suffered a horrible surgical mishap while undergoing what was probably an unnecessary lumbar fusion. One of the surgeons placed a screw to hold the fusion together, through a nerve going down into her right leg. He removed the screw in the operating room, but the damage was done. She awoke with severe right-leg pain and required a catheter to urinate. Her foot, part of her leg, the right half of her vagina, and rectum were numb.

Aside from a slight improvement in her urinary function, she remained as she had been on awakening. She also developed persistent and severe low-back pain. She had not worked at all for four months when she saw me, and was seriously thinking of declaring permanent disability. She was taking some minor painkillers, including nonanalgesic antidepressants, in a disorganized fashion, without apparent relief of pain or depression.

She consulted me for control of her pain and to try to get an explanation of what had really happened. No one had told her what had happened during surgery. After obtaining a series of radiological studies, I understood the damage incurred by the screw. I told her that she would not improve physically but didn't have to live with so much pain. She would need some form of pain medication for the rest of her life. I also told her I wanted to try to help her return to work if she, and her former employer, would work with me. She agreed and investigated the possibility of returning to work on some basis. The employer had been thrilled with her performance prior to her mishap and was willing to work with her disability as much as possible.

After a few weeks, we had worked out the basis for a complicated drug regimen, and over the next two months fine-tuned it, controlling most of the side effects well enough for her to work. She had increased difficulty urinating and became quite constipated on the drugs, and was so sleepy she couldn't read a book without dozing—even a good book.

Her nerve injury continued to work against her. It had damaged some of the nerves used for bowel and bladder function. Drugs, especially narcotics and tricyclics, can also interfere with these functions. So I stopped the tricyclics, altered her narcotic regimen, improved the medication that controlled her bowel function, added a second drug for her neuropathic leg pain, and performed a surgical procedure on her that dramatically relieved a significant portion of her terrible back pain. This allowed us to reduce her narcotics by 40 percent.

A urologist was able to help her void better with some new medication. We effectively combated her residual sleepiness with Ritalin, an amphetamine. I remember how she greeted me four weeks after the pain-relieving procedure, after she had been living on her new drug regimen for a while. She had tears of joy because something had been done to help her. However, in spite of the good outcome of the medication and the surgery, she had become depressed about her disability.

She was a beautiful woman who now walked with a cane, lived in some degree of chronic pain, and wasn't sure she could ever enjoy sexual relations again—or, for that matter, if she would ever be asked out by a man again. I don't know what I would do in her shoes, so I suggested she see a psychiatrist to help her with the emotional hurdles. I am pleased that with a reasonable amount of pain medication, some psychotherapy, and medication for depression, she went back to work as a nurse practitioner three days a week, enjoying the challenge of her job. She obviously still carries a lot of physical and psychological baggage around, but she is stronger and carries it more easily. These results are not exceptional. I had simply done my job, the task of any physician who treats pain.

KEY POINTS
About Medication for Pain

- Pain can be minimized even if its underlying cause cannot be cured.

- Taking narcotics to control pain does not lead to addiction.

- Taking pain medication does not mean you are a weakling.

- The sooner pain is controlled or ended, the less medication is required. Most doctors do not prescribe adequate pain medication, which means patients suffer unnecessarily.

4

Headaches from Hell and Other Pains Above the Neck

When the head aches all members partake of the pains.

—MIGUEL DE CERVANTES

Headaches are one of the most common reasons for seeking medical attention. Most of us have had at least one headache, and one in four of us is plagued with chronic or severe recurrent headaches. Moreover, the percentage of those suffering with various types of headaches varies little across various Western European cultures. Some headaches, such as migraines, vary by sex and ethnic group, however, suggesting a strong biological and genetic component.

Headaches can be caused by some underlying disease process—such as brain tumors, hemorrhages around or in the brain, meningitis, increased or decreased pressure within the spinal fluid bathing the brain, and of course less serious illnesses such as a flu. However, 90 percent of headaches are not associated with any particular disease.

Head and face pain arises from various pain-sensitive structures within the bones, dura (covering of the brain or spinal cord), muscles, joints, vessels, sinuses, eyes, ears, teeth, throat, and nerves of the head, jaw, and neck.

Like any other pain, headache may be test-negative by conventional criteria or may arise from serious recognizable problems, such as abnormally dilated masses of blood vessels within the brain that require complicated medical or surgical treatment. Certain tumors, including some cancers, can cause head and face pain. If you have persistent head or face pain, don't let your doctor—or anyone else—treat you without first obtaining a high-quality MRI of your brain and, if needed, lower skull, face, and neck. You need to rule out possible life-threatening causes of the pain.

Migraines: Stop Pounding on My Head

Migraines occur in at least 16 percent of American women and 7 percent of men. They are more common in Caucasians than African-Americans and less common in Asians than either, pointing to a genetic factor. Seventy percent of migraine patients have a family history of the disease, another clue that genetics plays a strong role in migraine. Migraines peak between the ages of twenty-five and fifty-five—the most productive years. Over the last twenty years, migraines appear to have increased by at least 60 percent in the United States, suggesting either better diagnosis or that we are paying the piper for our frantic lifestyle. We really don't know why more patients are suffering from these headaches.

About twenty-three million Americans suffer from severe migraines and 25 percent of them experience four or more severe attacks monthly. One-third are so severely disabled they need bed rest during an attack. You can tell where we are going—this is one expensive headache. Annual costs for lost productivity in the United States due to migraines range from $1.2 billion to $17.2 billion. Moreover, about 50 percent of the migraine population—the most disabled—accounts for 90 percent of lost workdays.

The scenario below describes the tragedy of the headache. The scene starts as the headless horseman, trotting up from behind, seeks his unknowing victim, walking calmly down toward the end of a steep canyon, with no escape. The "victim" experiences strange feelings walking up the canyon—fatigue and anxiety, for no apparent reason. These are followed by visions of blinking lights or flashbulbs igniting. However, the victim, not having learned the full scenario of migraine, glances uneasily over her shoulder, but is still unaware of the horseman inexorably approaching in the darkness.

Suddenly, out of the darkness, the horseman gallops forth, huge, raised sword in hand, his fierce steed snorting as his hooves pound the ground underneath in a dreadful, unrelenting rhythm. The poor victim, screaming in anticipation of the headache of the century, is swiftly beheaded. Then the horseman turns his well-schooled mount around in an elegant pirouette and gallops back out of the canyon, down a short, windy road to the well lit, bustling, noisy shop of a sadistic blacksmith. The horseman throws the head to the smithy, who begins pounding his horseshoes on it.

This tragedy may be played in four acts.

Act I. This devilish headache is often preceded an hour or a day in advance by a strange feeling, or "prodrome." This may be associated with lack of pep, increased irritability (wait until the headache strikes if you want to see irritability), or cravings—like for a delightful chocolate truffle or even a Snickers bar, depending on the victim's fancy and pocketbook.

Act II. While they are a minority, 20 percent of migraine sufferers get a warning that we call an aura, which includes problems with vision, such as the perception of a cluster of flashbulbs flashing. However, these auras may also include areas of numbness or tingling around the lips or in the fingers or supersensitive skin. Rarely, some people may feel as if they are in a different place or time, like Alice in Wonderland. You should be getting the idea that this is no ordinary headache, but a phenomenon affecting the whole brain. The headache usually comes after this aura, although it may appear before or during this early phase. Specialists often miss the diagnosis of migraine by insisting on an aura, which in fact is seen only in a minority of migraine sufferers.

Act III. The headache itself is usually associated with throbbing pain, although aching can occur. I remember seeing as a child a commercial for Anacin showing a hammer banging an anvil. That's a migraine throbbing. The pain may be on one side (in about 60 percent of cases) or on both sides. It also can switch sides. These headaches increase in intensity as they progress. As if this isn't bad enough, gradually nausea, occasional vomiting, and excessive sensitivity to light and noise follow. During this time, sufferers may have difficulty concentrating and thinking clearly. They may experience sore muscles. The headache worsens with physical activity or jostling the head around, so patients want to lie down in a quiet dark room. These headaches last for four hours to—believe it or not—*three days*. I'd rather be beheaded with a dull sword! Occasionally, the headaches may persist even longer.

Act IV. After the headache stops, the patient gets her head put back on—well, in a manner of speaking. She enters a period called the "postdrome," where she feels hungover. She still may not think quite clearly and still have some stomach upset as well as muscle ache. She also may feel elated—not, apparently, for the reason you would expect, joy at the end of the torture session, but because of chemical changes in the brain.

What are these changes? Will the real horseman and blacksmith please stand up? Of course, if migraine were truly understood, it wouldn't be such a costly burden to patients and society. The aura, and maybe the prodrome, of migraine are associated with a depression or inhibition of the brain's cortex. This explains the strange feelings patients have. What causes this depression is possibly some trigger deep in the vital part at the base of the brain, a complex area that controls the activity of a host of neurochemical systems in the brain.

What triggers the trigger? All sorts of things, and they don't necessarily apply to all patients or even to the same patient all the time. However, alcohol (especially red wine), emotional letdown after stressful periods (a great reward for finishing final exams), menstruation, ovulation, the Pill, too little or too much sleep, ingesting certain foods (chocolate, certain cheeses, MSG, processed meats), and changes in the weather or sun exposure can all bring on migraines. I have seldom met a female migraine sufferer who doesn't get headaches from a St.-Emilion, a French Bordeaux made primarily from the merlot grape.

Migraine pain appears to result from activation or increased activity of the structures subserving the trigeminal nerve in the brain and the blood vessels it supplies. The three components of the headache are dilation of vessels within the brain, inflammation around these vessels, and increased electrical and chemical activity in the trigeminal pain-processing system. The blood-vessel distension, worse with each heartbeat, and vessel inflammation are thought to explain the terrible throbbing that migraine sufferers experience when they move their heads during attacks. The neurotransmitter serotonin is thought to play a vital role in causing migraine, and the most effective drugs for controlling severe migraine and its side effects manipulate this transmitter, or, more precisely, the various receptors to which it binds.

Binding of various drugs to different types of serotonin receptors may help prevent migraines from getting worse, treat ongoing headaches, and block the nausea and vomiting associated with these headaches.

Treatment for Migraine

There are various new drugs—the triptans—which bind to one type of serotonin receptor and in so doing achieve excellent control of *all* the various symptoms of the migraine, not just the headache, with far fewer side effects than older drugs. They may be somewhat useful even when a headache is advanced. These drugs reduce the pain of migraine by constricting the dilated blood vessels and reducing the inflammation around them.

Triptans include sumatriptan (Imitrex), zolmitriptan (Zomig), naratriptan (Amerge), and rizatriptan (Maxalt). The first comes in injectable, nasal spray, and pill forms, and the others only in pill form. Injectable Imitrex helps more than 80 percent of patients quickly, and is the most effective. The highly beneficial effect of the drug is seen only if it is taken early during the headache. Taken at the height of the attack, it may relieve the migraine symptoms in about 35 percent of patients.

When taken properly, Imitrex is particularly useful in treating severe migraines. Amerge, which is quite long-acting, works better on moderate migraines and during menstrual periods. During a migraine, which may cause gastrointestinal disturbance including nausea and vomiting, oral medication in tablet form is not always well digested. Maxalt is interesting in that it may be dissolved as a wafer under the tongue—a boon to those who tolerate pills poorly during migraines and for those who can't take pills without water. Maxalt may be the most effective oral triptan.

The older drugs, such as those derived from ergotamine, caffeine (Cafergot) and dihydroergotamine (DHE-45), also constrict dilated blood vessels, but cause more side effects, including nausea. Other drugs, such as NSAIDs, are helpful in reducing pain and inflammation in moderately severe migraines. Corticosteroids may also be used in short courses. Narcotics may be used to relieve pain in severe migraine, if nothing else works well. Drugs to fight nausea may also be useful.

Botox injections. Recently, a nerve toxin involved in botulism poisoning, called botulinum toxin or Botox, has been injected in small amounts into the scalp muscles of migraine patients, over the sites of the pain, with quite good results. In these small doses the toxin is quite safe and has no significant side effects. The toxin relaxes the muscles for months and may be reinjected at several-month intervals. What is interesting about this is that by controlling scalp-muscle contraction, a reaction to the headache and the pain it causes, you can better control the headache. Presumably, the injection reduces the pain from the tight scalp muscles, reducing the overall painful input to the trigeminal system of migraine patients—a system that is already in overdrive. Pain may feed itself, and this injection may block a self-perpetuating cycle of headache–muscle tightness–headache and so on. Logically, in terms of theory, this type of injection should also relieve tension headaches, described below.

Keeping Migraines at Bay

If you have frequent migraines, the trick is to avoid the headaches completely with medication. Tricyclic antidepressants may be effective in reducing the severity and frequency of the horseman's visits. Drugs like Prozac and its cousins, however, are not effective in preventing migraine. But since patients with severe migraine can become depressed, these drugs can still help them, just as the drugs are used to treat depression associated with neuropathic pain.

A class of heart or blood pressure drugs known as beta blockers is also helpful. Inderal is an example of this kind of drug. Two anticonvulsants, Neurontin and Depakote, may also help control frequent migraine. Women with migraine around the menstrual period may benefit from reducing body water by using a water pill, like hydrochlorthiazide, for about five days before menstruation. This also helps PMS (premenstrual syndrome) symptoms.

Finally, biofeedback may help some people reduce the severity and frequency of headaches. On a purely anecdotal basis, I have seen some patients who have also improved after acupuncture. A moderate and consistent lifestyle with regular mealtimes, exercise, and sleep routines may help keep the migraines away. Remember, moderation is hard to achieve in our fast-paced society.

If nothing seems to work for you, then see a headache specialist before the disease destroys you and your life.

CLUSTER HEADACHES: GET THAT ICE PICK OUT OF MY EYE!

Unlike migraines, the cluster headache favors men. This type of headache is ferocious in its severity, but fortunately is far less common than migraines, affecting only about four hundred thousand men and ninety thousand women in the United States. It usually strikes patients starting at around age twenty-five and tends to subside by age fifty. Unlike migraines, it tends not to run in families or particular ethnic groups, suggesting it may not have a strong genetic influence.

There are two forms of cluster headache, the episodic and the chronic. Episodic headaches, which affect 80 percent of patients with this disease, usually occur in clusters—thus the name—over a period of several weeks to three months. They occur every day or several times a day, at about the same hour. They last fifteen minutes to several hours. Then they disappear, not to return for months or even years. The chronic form doesn't disappear.

The headache usually begins quickly, with excruciating pain in or around one eye but not both. However, either eye can be affected in any headache. Patients describe pain vividly as feeling like an ice pick in the eye. The pain is usually sharp and constant, but can involve throbbing sensations as well. The headache is characterized by far more than pain. Patients *may* have redness of the covering of the eye, tearing, a stuffy or runny nose, sweating of the forehead and face, a constricted pupil, and a drooping or puffy eyelid. So you see, this headache may resemble an excruciating allergy. It has nothing to do with allergies, however. It may be triggered by alcohol, but only during a cluster.

No one really knows what causes the cluster headache. One theory is that, like migraines, it results from blood-vessel dilation, but most researchers feel that the blood-vessel abnormalities are not the root cause. Another theory proposes an intrinsic brain abnormality. This is supported by the fact that these patients have a disruption of their biorhythms during their headaches. Finally, there is a theory that invokes some abnormality of the carotid arteries delivering blood to the brain.

Treatment for Cluster Headaches

Treatments for cluster headaches are thought to relieve the pain by constricting blood vessels that are presumably dilated and possibly inflamed. Remember this from Migraine 101? So Imitrex and ergotamine drugs are useful to treat an acute attack—to remove that ice pick. To keep it out, various drugs may be used, including a particular NSAID called indomethacin (Indocin), short courses of steroids, lithium (also used to treat manic-depressives), and calcium channel blockers, which control blood pressure by dilating vessels.

In certain cases, one of two surgical procedures may be performed with quite good results. In the first, the sphenopalatine ganglion, a location of nerve cells next to the nose and under the eye, may be lesioned, using the radiofrequency technique, with approximately 60 to 85 percent of patients deriving benefit. Similarly, lesions of the pain-carrying fibers of the trigeminal nerve have been effective in close to 70 percent of cases.

TENSION HEADACHES: PLEASE LOOSEN THE HEADBAND!

By far the most common headache, occurring in about 35 percent of adults and 45 percent of all headache patients, is the two-sided, pressing, aching headache seen on television. You know, the one where the patient holds the forehead and complains: "I have a headache." It is annoying but not disabling like the last two monsters. It also has none of the complicated problems associated with the other headaches. It can last from less than an hour to all week and definitely wears its victim down. There appear to be no triggers for this type of headache—you can eat and drink whatever you feel like and still get it.

It is thought to be due to muscle contraction over the scalp, a type of myofascial pain. However, patients with this problem often have preexisting depression and anxiety, possibly worsened by poorly controlled headaches. They may also have an abnormal pain-processing system.

Treatment for Tension Headaches

Treatment of these headaches involves use of muscle relaxants, tricyclic antidepressants, and other painkillers. However, using pain relievers like NSAIDs or preparations like Fiorinal (caffeine, a barbiturate, and aspirin) or Fioricet (substitute the aspirin in Fiorinal with acetaminophen) more than once weekly on a regular basis invites a worse problem—rebound headaches (see below).

Obviously, on a bad week you can certainly exceed one pill. The trick then is not to take any headache remedies for the next week or so. Also, remember that eventually any aspirin-containing compound may catch up with your stomach, and any acetaminophen-containing compound (like Tylenol) may damage your liver in high enough doses, if you're foolish enough to abuse either one of them. Nonpharmacological methods, such as biofeedback and relaxation techniques (such as meditation), may also help (see chapter 2).

REBOUND HEADACHES: THE CURE IS KILLING ME

Sometimes physicians' ministrations create their own problems, as bad as if not worse than the disease being treated. Rebound headaches are a

dreadful form of headache caused by taking too much headache medicine. It is most common in patients with tension and migraine headaches.
I know, you can't win and you can't break even. It's bad enough to be
cursed with these headaches, but now the treatment is poisoning you.

Most headache remedies can cause these headaches—the Fioricet-
type compounds, narcotics, and even over-the-counter medications.
One additional contributing cause of these headaches is excessive use
of caffeine. Remember, caffeine exists not just in delightful home-
ground espresso, but in all those caffeinated soft drinks (a dreadful
substitute for fine coffee, freshly brewed tea, or a great cup of the
finest Dutch cocoa, in my humble opinion).

You can see how the headache victim becomes akin to a raving drug
addict, although these rebound headaches are less a form of addiction than a form of tolerance (see chapter 3). Patients have severe
headaches, take medicine that helps them, and they feel better—until
the headache returns and the cycle starts all over again. Soon enough,
the headaches become more frequent or more severe, and more medication is needed to put them back to sleep. Eventually, you are off to
the headache-drug races again and the headaches win. Mephistopheles
comes to claim Faust. The seductive salutary effect of headache remedies can be such as to cause rebound headaches within three weeks.

POST-TRAUMATIC HEADACHES

A blow to the head can change your life forever in many ways, including bringing on headaches from which you may suffer chronically. Why
head trauma may bring on migraines, for example, is not clear. Maybe
those who develop them after trauma were genetically predisposed and
ongoing head and neck pain in the weeks following the trauma may
somehow have sensitized the trigeminal system. One kind of headache
that may arise following trauma can be controlled quite well, if not
cured (see the section on head trauma, p.78).

Cervicogenic Headaches

Cervicogenic headaches are triggered or perpetuated by inflammation
of or trauma to pain-generating structures such as muscles, ligaments,
tendons, disks, facets (see chapter 6), or nerves in and around the cervical spine (the part of the spine in the neck). The most likely source
of persistent cervicogenic headaches, barring any significant cervical-
spine instability or other potential surgical problem, is the upper three

cervical facets, the joints that stabilize the spine. A fall, a whiplash injury, a blow to the head in boxing, an object falling on the head from above—all can cause these headaches. Arthritis can cause them in older patients.

These headaches may be one-sided or two-sided. They may be aching, sharp, or throbbing. Cervicogenic headaches often awaken patients or exist when they wake up, and may or may not get worse during the day. They are often worsened by looking up or to the side (or sides) where the headache is. Although they are often associated with complaints referable to the neck, patients may simply complain of pain in the front of the head, without describing neck pain or pain at the back or side of the head. For this reason, cervicogenic headaches are confused with some form of headache not related to neck problems and are not diagnosed properly. However, careful physical examination usually reveals tenderness over the sides or back of the neck, as well as pain when the patient assumes various neck positions.

There is a poor correlation between patients' symptoms and radiological findings on MRIs, CAT scans, and plain X rays of the head and neck, which is why these patients are often written off as malingerers or psychiatric cases. Unfortunately, some of these patients may well become psychiatric cases because of ongoing depression and anxiety brought on by their chronic, poorly understood, and ineffectually treated pain. This in turn may result in a complex patient, difficult to treat and rehabilitate.

When to See a Headache Specialist

A good internist—even better, a good neurologist—can treat most headaches. However, if you have headaches that are seriously disturbing your life because of their frequency and severity or the miserable side effects of the medicine, go see a good headache specialist—a compassionate, imaginative expert at treating headaches. These are usually neurologists with a special interest in headaches. Because of this special interest, they may be able to obtain and give you new drugs before they hit the market. Given the rate of advancement in producing new and effective drugs for migraines, getting a drug early may be beneficial. You may find a new drug that really works, reducing your suffering by months.

My own interest in headache treatment is utilizing interventional procedures to help control headaches that do not respond to medication. This kind of approach applies to no more than 20 percent of all headache patients. The most likely patients for me to treat are those with cervicogenic headaches or cluster headaches. A small percentage of patients with the diagnosis of migraine or tension headache may have pain that is referred to the head from the neck. The point is, some of these patients who do not respond to any drugs well, and begin to see their lives trickle down through the sieves of disability, dysfunction, depression, and anger, should at least be evaluated for other treatments that may benefit them. This is especially true for treatments that can be given, or pain-relieving procedures that can be performed, with a good record of long-term success and little risk of a bad outcome. On that basis, they are certainly worth considering.

The Woman Who Loved Roller Coasters

A fifty-year-old Chicago woman had chronic daily headaches on both sides of her head for nine years following a wild roller-coaster ride during which she had suffered a whiplashlike injury. She *really* liked roller coasters. (To each his—or her—own!) She had had no headaches until that amusement-park adventure. Her son had suggested she consult with me after seeing me on a national television show in which I demonstrated the utility of radiofrequency lesioning in the relief of various pain syndromes. This technique uses highly controlled heat, delivered precisely to a discrete area, to destroy selectively the nerves carrying pain impulses to the brain. The woman and her husband, a psychiatrist, came to see if I could help her.

Over the years, she suffered from her symptoms and became disabled. During the almost-daily episodic flare-up of her headaches—lasting many hours—she would spend much of her time in the house, frequently resorting to resting in a quiet, dark room, taking her medication, and waiting for it to work. She had been a patient in several major headache clinics and was currently under the care of a neurologist who could offer her only a combination of several drugs with a modest beneficial effect. The woman had already tried a total of 150 different medications for headache relief with minimal to modest effect.

In Chicago, she recently had inquired about and been turned down for a radiofrequency procedure to alleviate her head pain. The physician in question felt her particular situation didn't merit any radiofrequency procedure. He also implied that he was reluctant to perform this kind of procedure on her neck under any circumstances. What she was looking for was a cervical radiofrequency facet neurotomy. A what? In this procedure, the nerves to the facets, or supporting joints, in the neck are destroyed or lesioned using radiofrequency technique—a means of applying heat, in an exquisitely precise fashion, for the purpose of selectively destroying (lesioning) the little nerves that transmit sensation, including pain, from the facet joints to the brain.

I ordered MRI and CAT scans of her cervical spine. They revealed minor arthritic changes, but nothing worthy of any form of spinal surgery. On examination, pressure over the mid-to-upper facets on both sides of her neck revealed tenderness. Deep pressure applied to the uppermost facets elicited head pain over the front of her skull, above her eyebrows.

I reasoned that, in part, her headaches might be connected to the pain in her neck, which originated from her facets. Somehow, minor trauma to her cervical facets occurred at the time of her whiplashlike injury, during her roller-coaster ride nine years earlier. This trauma had led to a chronic pain condition, which referred to her head from her neck. Her headaches also had a migrainous quality. I also told her that some of the medication she was taking for the control of her head pain may have produced rebound headaches, and insisted that she taper herself off the medication as a condition of being my patient.

To determine whether lesioning the nerves to her facets would be effective, I evaluated her with diagnostic nerve blocks of the nerves supplying the facets on both sides of her neck. She had excellent relief of her pain from these blocks. Nevertheless, she was apprehensive about undergoing radiofrequency lesioning of the nerves in question. I suggested she contact some of my former patients, which she did. Her fears were allayed by the success and minimal discomfort experienced by my other patients with similar complaints and treatment.

She decided to undergo lesioning of her cervical facets, which was accomplished without difficulty in two stages. She recovered uneventfully from the procedures and has been virtually free of headache and has not required any headache medication in the year following her two-week recovery from the procedure. She wants to go to Disney World. I told her to enjoy herself but not ride any roller coasters while she's down there. It is nice to see her get back into a fuller life.

ATYPICAL FACIAL PAIN

The name alone tells you anyone who has this is in trouble. They suffer from a problem that doesn't fit into any category that is understood. There is no known cause for this problem, so those that suffer are often given short shrift because the pain is test-negative and its victims are women, whose test-negative pain is often regarded as being emotional. This is a facial pain disorder usually seen in women who are anxious or depressed. If uncontrolled, their pain may worsen their psychological symptoms. The pain is chronic, deep, and unaffected by facial or head movements. Patients with this disorder often undergo multiple dental and facial surgeries with no benefit other than to keep the economy moving. The pain is not easily treated with most pain medications. Small doses of tricyclics, such as Pamelor, may be helpful.

These patients require a thorough evaluation by a compassionate, skilled physician who takes them seriously enough to look for other causes of their pain—disorders that may be treated more effectively than this atypical type of pain.

Psychological Treatment

Psychotherapy may help these patients for two reasons. First, they have a problem that is depressing—they are in pain and nobody knows why or can really help them. We may find one day that this is like many other painful disorders—that there is a very good basis for it that we don't yet recognize. Second, allegiance with a supportive psychiatrist, or a nonmedical mental-health professional if no medication is needed, may help these patients avoid spending money and time and taking the risks of just one more facial or dental surgical procedure.

JAWS: TEMPOROMANDIBULAR JOINT SYNDROME (TMJ)

What exactly is dysfunction of the temporomandibular (jaw) joint? The major complaint in patients with this problem is pain around the joint, which spreads to the temple, part of the face, and the muscles of the neck and scalp. Pain may involve one or both sides of the face. Chewing increases pain and the mouth cannot open fully. In addition, there may also be a clicking as the jaw moves. There may be right or left deviation of the lower jaw noted on examination by a dentist or a specialist familiar with this disorder. But TMJ dysfunction often, not always, is associated with no identifiable abnormality on appropriate X-ray studies. Therefore, it is often test-negative. Focal areas of tenderness in painful muscles (myofascial pain with trigger points) in the area of pain may exist.

Doctors believe the disorder is caused by muscle tension from clenching the jaws and grinding the teeth, especially at night. This may be caused by anxiety and depression.

Poor alignment of the biting mechanism may be caused by or cause arthritic changes in the joints. Other causes of TMJ dysfunction include trauma (a punch in the jaw), joint degeneration due to aging, and other forms of arthritis.

Early on in my practice, a twenty-year-old man came to me complaining of some pain on the left side of his neck and terrible headaches over the left forehead that were worse in the morning. (This is typical of headaches that originate in the neck. As a patient twists and turns during sleep, they aggravate their neck problems.) He had already been evaluated for one type of one-sided chronic headache (not due to soreness in the neck) that responds to a particular nonsteroidal medication—indomethacin—but had no effect on him.

I examined the man and concluded that his pain might be from painful facets in the upper-left neck. After a diagnostic block of the nerves to those joints, to my surprise he said he still had the headache. This told me that either I was wrong in my diagnosis or the block was somehow technically unsuccessful. I actually repeated the same procedure right then and there, and still there was no relief of his pain. His slight chronic neck pain was gone, but he had the headache. So I figured something else might be causing these primarily one-sided headaches.

As he got up from the procedure he complained that the way he had been lying made his jaw hurt. The procedure was performed under guidance of a CAT scanner; I thought his painful jaw was related to the way he was positioned on the CAT table. I asked him to open and close his mouth. He was barely able to open it, so I attempted to force it open gently. This caused pain in the temporomandibular joints, especially on the left—the side of his headache. When I pressed on these joints gently, he felt considerable local pain. I concluded that his head and possibly even his neck pain came from his seemingly dysfunctional temporomandibular joints. I sent him to a dentist who specialized in this area, who confirmed my diagnosis. The patient had referred head and neck pain from severe degeneration of the TMJ joints—a finding later demonstrated on the special X rays and MRI obtained by the dentist.

My patient was annoyed that I hadn't looked at his mouth before evaluating his neck with nerve blocks. He was justified, to some extent. I had underestimated the powerful role TMJ pain may play in certain headaches. However, the dentist told me that the negative results from the blocks helped him focus his diagnosis and treatment on the temporomandibular joints.

I learned a lot from this complicated patient. Ever since then, whenever someone comes to me complaining of head and certain neck pains, especially in the front or side of the head and side of the neck, I examine the jaws.

Treatment of TMJ Syndrome

TMJ dysfunction is usually treated with drugs to control anxiety or depression, muscle relaxants, NSAIDs, physical therapy, bite plates (preventing teeth grinding at night), and behavioral therapy. I like to prescribe a low dose of the tricylic antidepressant Pamelor, occasional use of a powerful Valium-like drug (Klonopin) at night, bite plates, and trigger-point injections of affected muscles. For the latter two forms of treatment, I send the patient to a dentist specializing in the nonsurgical treatment of this disease. Surgery on the joints is rarely indicated, but is too often performed, with poor results.

HEAD TRAUMA

Head trauma serves to illustrate the complicated interaction between physical and psychological pain and dysfunction. It is not difficult to understand how someone who was in a bad car accident, ended up with a skull fracture and a broken vertebral body (see chapter 6) in the neck, and was in a coma for three weeks may have prolonged head and neck pain and difficulty thinking. It would not be surprising if these problems were permanent. However, even minor head trauma can cause permanent pain and cognitive disability.

For example, a concussion is a transient impairment of brain function, commonly seen when a boxer is "stunned" but not knocked unconscious. We now know that repeated blows to the head eventually may cause enough permanent brain damage to result in *dementia pugilistica*, or dementia due to repeated blows to the head from fighting seen especially in older boxers.

One episode of relatively minor head trauma can lead to test-negative physical pain, dysfunction in thinking, paying attention, concentrating, calculating, and remembering; insomnia; loss of sexual drive; and eventual psychological disability and socioeconomic decline. Why some patients develop these long-term aftereffects from minor trauma and others do not isn't clear. We also don't know why some people develop prolonged pain following a whiplash injury and others do not. Cultural and psychological factors may play a role in how patients experience and report pain. Nevertheless, chronic pain and disability following minor trauma are real and, sadly for the patients suffering with these problems, are misunderstood by many physicians and attorneys and by the insurance industry.

Doctors must treat the physical pain as well as the brain dysfunction and psychological problems in order to rehabilitate anyone with cognitive dysfunction. Unfortunately, persistent cognitive difficulties following even minor head trauma may be a source of major, permanent disability. Following minor head trauma, some patients really do sustain some degree of brain damage—a physical problem. This damage may not be severe enough (or big enough) to show up on our sophisticated MRIs and the like, but is enough to cause these patients to perform suboptimally on psychological tests.

Examinations of the brains of people who developed cognitive side effects associated with a major concussion, but who died of other causes, have shown microscopic physical changes in the concussed brains. It is not surprising that minor-head-trauma patients cannot always be totally rehabilitated or cured. This is especially true for many holding intellectually or technically oriented jobs in modern urban society.

The Accountant Who Got Hit in the Head with a Briefcase

One morning as Jeanne, a thirty-seven-year-old accountant, got up from her bus seat, a ten-pound briefcase fell from the overhead rack and hit her on the back of the head. Although she was stunned, she remained conscious and went to work. Over the next few hours she felt aching pain in both sides of her neck and head. Over the next few days, when she moved her head a certain way, she felt dizzy. She also had trouble concentrating and was noticeably irritable. After several weeks, she developed pains on both sides of her neck going into her shoulders. She went to her local medical doctor, who obtained X rays of her skull and neck that indicated no abnormality. She was told to buy an over-the-counter nonsteroidal drug and to return to work in a few days.

Over the course of a few months, Jeanne's head and neck pain caused significant pain several times a week. Headaches radiated from her upper neck and skull base to her forehead and were worse when she looked up or turned her head to either side. This pain often woke her in the middle of the night or occurred in the morning when she

awoke. Some were severe, lasting as long as a day, and were very difficult to relieve, even with prescription medicine that she began taking.
Jeanne was often dizzy, had difficulty thinking and remembering, was
often irritable, and had crying spells. She and her husband began to
argue more and to confront ongoing problems in their marriage. She
soon became depressed.

After four months, Jeanne was placed on temporary disability. She
went to an attorney to help her prepare to seek monetary compensa-
tion for her injuries. The attorney sent her to a neurologist who examined her and obtained MRIs of her brain and neck. These studies
revealed no problems with her brain and only some age-related degeneration in her facets and disks.

The neurologist diagnosed her as having various aftereffects from
the blow to the head—headache, myofascial (muscle-related) pain,
damage to her equilibrium system, mental changes due to her presumed concussion, and depression due to her reaction to her general
disability. He prescribed an antidepressant and told her to try to go
back to work. The antidepressant seemed to worsen her headaches
and made her more irritable. On her own, she stopped the medication
and actually slightly improved, soon returning to the same rather miserable state she had been in before taking the antidepressant. The objective medical findings led her attorney to conclude she did not have
a strong case and that she could obtain no more than a few thousand
dollars.

Six months after her accident Jeanne came to me. Her dizziness was
better, but still persistent. Her neck pain and headaches continued to be
severe and her depression appeared to be significant. I agreed with her
earlier diagnoses, but I felt that her headache originated in her neck,
the result of inflammation following trauma to the upper and middle
cervical facets. My diagnosis was based on Jeanne's history, which included a whiplash component; the head and neck pain that was elicited
when she looked up or to the side when I pressed the muscles over the
facets; and the worsening of her pain during or just after sleep.

Unlike back pain, which is related to weight bearing, neck pain is
often worse with tossing and turning as we go in and out of dream
sleep. Sleeping on our backs, with the head facing up and the spine relatively straight (not bent up over an overstuffed pillow), is the best position to limit neck pain and the headaches related to neck pain.
Unfortunately, most of us sleep on our side or, worse yet, on our stomach, with the neck turned at a near ninety-degree angle to the side

from the usual face-forward position, stressing the neck structures considerably (see chapter 2).

Also, in my experience, patients who have a whiplash injury, with pain in the neck, head, or low back persisting over several months without a good radiological basis to explain their symptoms (such as bone displacement, fracture, or disk herniation), usually have a significant degree of facet-related pain. Myofascial pain (see chapter 5) may accompany the above but is usually a response to the underlying pain. Discogenic pain (emanating from degenerated disks; see chapter 6) may coexist with the facet-related pain, but is less common. For these reasons, I decided eventually to evaluate the role her facets played in her ongoing painful disability.

However, Jeanne's symptoms were so general that I thought she needed a team approach. I sent her to a famous rehabilitation facility, with experience in treating victims of major and minor head trauma. She saw a psychologist to help her sort out her emotions and a rehabilitation physician who specialized in treating equilibrium disturbance following head injury. This form of rehabilitation required repetitive neck turning, which was impeded by her pain. I was asked to treat her neck pain in order for her rehabilitation to proceed.

First, I had to diagnose, with relative certainty, the neck structures generating her neck and possibly head pain based on her history, the unimpressive radiological studies, and physical examination. On a day she had particularly bad head and neck pain, I performed diagnostic nerve blocks on the nerves relaying pain messages to the brain from the sore facets in her neck. These blocks temporarily relieved her pain completely.

The robust effect of these blocks served to demonstrate several things. She cried after the block out of a sense of relief—relief from pain for the first time in months; relief that her pain might one day be eradicated or, at least, significantly improved; and relief that she really wasn't crazy. She had come to wonder if all her problems were due to the depression. She minimized the fact that her depression came on after she had developed chronic disabling symptoms that did not show up on tests and that were not thought to be serious by her doctors or lawyer. She recalled how her neurologist told her, "You should consider yourself lucky. Nothing is wrong with you. You just got banged up a bit and have overreacted to your problems."

The block also demonstrated that her pain was not truly "test-negative." Her pain or its basis was not visualized on a regular MRI, but the potential cause of her pain was testable by another method.

Admittedly, the use of nerve blocks to make diagnoses is fraught with potential problems. However, blocks may be used to support a clinical impression. Certainly, if the blocks did not relieve her pain, it would have been inappropriate to further treat the joints in her neck as major causes of her pain. Similar symptoms can result from painful disks in the neck, even without herniation or pressure on nerve roots. The disks would have been investigated by discography (see chapter 6) to determine if they caused her pain. Finally, even if these block-based tests had failed to elucidate the cause of her pain, I would maintain that her pain was quite real, but modern medicine was unable to understand it. "Test-negativity" may simply represent the diagnostic limitation of medicine and may not be a result of psychological dysfunction of our patients.

Because the blocks supported my clinical impression, I treated her cervical facet joints with radiofrequency lesioning of the nerves taking pain messages from the sore joints to the brain—cutting the lines of pain communication. This improved her head and neck pain by 90 percent and had a significant positive effect on her psychological situation. Her depression improved and she was able to work at her rehabilitation, diminishing her sense of equilibrium disturbance and learning what she could and could not accomplish mentally. She was one of the unfortunate patients who had long-term difficulties performing demanding higher mental functions following minor head trauma. Six months after treatment, she was able to return to work, but in a less demanding area of accounting.

Diagnosing the Aftereffects of Head Trauma

Jeanne's case demonstrates the difficulty of proper diagnosis. Her MRIs did not show any physical damage from being hit on the head. Yet she had developed long-standing, disabling head, neck, and shoulder pain, intermittent dizziness, difficulty with concentrating, irritability, and depression. Could she have been using the accident as an excuse—consciously or unconsciously—to get out of a stressful job, to seek financial gain, or to deal, however inappropriately, with chronic problems in her marriage? After all, pain can be based on discomfort from the body or the mind, as discussed in chapter 1. Whether she was dealing with psychological or financial issues or not, most of her pain was physical, as demonstrated by the fact that 90 percent of it went away when the nerves to her painful facets were destroyed. She has remained vastly improved for over three years.

Because she had so many disabling symptoms, with both psychological and physical components, she needed a team of a neurologist, a psychologist, and a physical-medicine specialist to help get her proper treatment. In this case, the psychologist determined that her mental health was basically sound, despite the stress she was under. Her depression was a reaction to her disability and improved as her disability lessened, beginning with the significant diminution of her pain.

Unfortunately, many physicians who care for head-trauma victims, including neurologists, neurosurgeons, and physiatrists (rehabilitation physicians), are unaware of patterns of pain following trauma, including referred pain. In evaluating a headache patient, most physicians don't even examine two common causes of head pain—the neck and the temporomandibular or jaw joint. As Jeanne's story illustrates amply, X rays and even more sophisticated MRIs may not demonstrate which structures contribute significantly to the patient's pain symptoms. Unfortunately, anatomically test-negative pain is quite common and not taken seriously by the majority of physicians today, who are trained to find an objective basis for disease by commonly accepted criteria.

The diagnosis and treatment of significant psychological problems in any chronic pain patient is imperative in providing appropriate pain management. Admittedly, undertreated physical pain may worsen the psychological dimension of a chronic pain syndrome. However, many pain patients are overtreated by pain-management specialists—often with excessive use of strong medication and costly, possibly risky, unproven invasive procedures for symptoms with a strong psychological component.

Depression and anxiety are commonly found following head trauma. Any chronic loss of function, independence, or social status (all of which may be caused by chronic pain syndrome) engenders psychological pain of various types. Depression, anxiety, frustration, and dysfunctional behavior are likely in patients whose disabling symptoms are misunderstood or labeled psychological by their own physicians or financially insignificant by their attorneys. In turn, these psychological variables often worsen a patient's perception of pain.

Conversely, physiatrists, neurologists, psychiatrists, and psychologists treating head-trauma patients must familiarize themselves with post-traumatic painful conditions. When those conditions impair the rehabilitative process, patients must be referred to specialized consultants who can diagnose and treat various painful conditions quickly and effectively.

The above case illustrates that treating pain involves addressing the physical, psychological, and socioeconomic aspects of the patient's condition. An experienced, multidisciplinary staff, dealing with various aspects of the body and the mind, best accomplishes the rehabilitation of head-trauma victims.

KEY POINTS
About Head Pain

- Head pain is usually test-negative.

- Doctors (including those in training), other health-care professionals, and key insurance company personnel must all become more knowledgeable about the existence of test-negative pain disorders and how to better evaluate and treat patients with them.

- Understand that you are not necessarily crazy—at least not yet—because you suffer from certain kinds of pain that are poorly understood by an often ignorant, arrogant, or intolerant medical system.

- Find a headache specialist who is sufficiently intelligent, curious, courageous, and open-minded to push the envelope of what is known—and who will debunk inadequate explanations (no matter how popular); strive to understand the presently unexplainable, and treat, and even cure, a condition that many doctors may consider untreatable.

- Seek out physicians who can understand and help you—even if you may have to pay for this type of sophisticated, compassionate expertise out of pocket.

- There are new medications to treat headache more effectively with fewer side effects.

- Ask your doctor about minimally invasive surgical procedures that can be used judiciously to treat otherwise intractable pain.

5

Treating Painful Muscles, Bones, and Joints

For the aging person it is a duty and a necessity to give serious attention to himself.

—CARL JUNG

More than half of the American population suffers from muscle pain. At least one-third of us have this pain for more than eleven days, and 10 percent of us have chronic muscle pain for more than a hundred days. Approximately forty-three million people, or one in six Americans, have arthritis pain; two out of three sufferers are women. Women also lead the way with pain from osteoporosis.

That's a lot of pain!

MYOFASCIAL PAIN

The number of people with myofascial pain, also known as trigger-point pain, is unknown, but the problem appears to be common. *Myo* refers to muscles and *fascia* is a tough coating that envelops our muscles like Saran Wrap. Many people have had this type of pain at one time or other without knowing its name. Myofascial pain is a major reason for obtaining massage, chiropractic manipulation, and physical therapy.

Medical science has shown that structural problems, like broken bones, tumors, disk herniations, or damaged nerves, cause chronic pain. However, Dr. Janet Travell, who was known to the public as President Kennedy's physician, and her colleague D. G. Simons expressed a theory that muscles themselves cause pain from abnormalities in bundles of muscle fibers called trigger points.

Myofascial pain is characterized by small areas of muscle tenderness, which, when poked, cause severe pain, often associated with triggering a jump away from the poking finger. Thus the name "trigger point." The pain produced by this nasty, probing, examining finger involves both the localized trigger point as well as defined patterns of referred pain. For example, mysofascial pain from the buttock produces localized buttock soreness as well as referred pain down the leg that mimics sciatica. Pain from the muscles used in chewing produces local pain in the jaw and temple as well as referred pain in the side of the neck and the head.

Myofascial pain may involve either very small focal areas or larger regional body areas. Focal pain is a small area of tenderness, occasionally as small as a knot of less than an inch to a few inches in diameter. Regional pain is the whole low back or side of the thigh or area from the neck down to the lower shoulder blade. However, compared with fibromyalgia, a competing diagnosis, myofascial pain exists in discrete areas within which well-localized trigger points are scattered. There trigger points are less widespread over the body than the diffusely tender points of fibromyalgia (see page 90).

Myofascial pain occurs equally in both sexes and affects all ages. It is often associated with muscle stiffness and fatigue and may plague you while you are moving or at rest. However, don't mistake this pain for muscle tension, like a spasm or cramp, or for the diffuse soreness of the flu. It appears to be caused by several factors, most commonly overuse or overstretching of unconditioned muscles. It is a form of pain common to workaholics who sit in a poor posture for hours in front of computers and couch potatoes who spend hours dulling their brain with television while slowly crippling themselves. Weekend warriors abusing those sedentary bodies without sufficient warm-up are also prime candidates for myofascial pain. (See chapter 2 on ways to prevent some of this pain.)

Other medical problems can mimic or even cause myofascial pain, such as certain muscle injuries (tears), some systemic rheumatological diseases, and fibromyalgia, for example. Fibromyalgia can follow or coexist with myofascial pain. Even depression and anxiety can cause or exacerbate myofascial pain.

Old injuries like a damaged shoulder from high school basketball make myofascial pain more likely to occur. Underlying pain from the spinal disks and facet joints is often associated with myofascial pain in the muscles overlying the painful spinal structures. In most people with one-sided lumbar or low-back facet pain, myofascial pain of the buttock and upper thigh muscles is exceedingly common, as is bursitis of the covering of the hip joint. Unless all three sources of pain (facets, muscles, and bursa) are treated, you will not get better. Muscles supplied by nerves pinched or compressed by herniated disks can also develop myofascial pain superimposed on that of the pinched nerve.

Diagnosis of Myofascial Pain
Myofascial pain is often test-negative. There are no X-ray or electrical diagnostic tests that can confirm the diagnosis. Examining the trigger points under a microscope reveals no consistent abnormality, so the diagnosis is purely clinical—based on your history and physical examination—especially when it comes to finding the trigger points that cause pain.

Unfortunately, many physicians consider this pain not terribly significant. For a few days, it may be annoying. If it lingers for several months, and results in significant deterioration of your lifestyle, and if you feel you are stuck with a disbelieving doctor, find another who will determine why you have persistent pain.

Treatment of Myofascial Pain
Noninvasive treatments include hot or cold packs, drugs (nonsteroidals or antidepressants), TENS (see chapter 2), acupuncture, and ultrasound applied to the overlying skin. These treatments may be used together if necessary. Here are some of the most common ways to treat this condition.

Trigger-Point Therapy. Injecting a local anesthetic into trigger points of tight muscles may relieve pain and return a sore muscle to normal functioning. Similar relief could be gained by dry needling (inserting a needle into the trigger point) or injecting saline (sterile salt water). These procedures, however, are more painful than injecting local anesthetics. There have been no well-controlled studies of trigger-point therapy for low-back or limb pain. Nevertheless, it is widely used.

Spray and stretch is a successful procedure that involves spraying a coolant over the skin overlying trigger points, followed by massaging or stretching the painful muscle. Since the spray-and-stretch procedure is less invasive than the trigger-point injections, it may be tried first.

Botox injection is the new kid on the block. This technique involves injection of a minuscule amount of a nerve toxin (see chapter 4). Used for medical purposes, this toxin actually causes a mild, isolated muscle weakness (not paralysis), lasting two to six months, providing long-term relaxation of trigger points and sustained relief from myofascial pain. Botox injections are an exciting therapy because of the sustained effect. However, Botox is expensive and, when used inappropriately, can cause excessive—albeit transient—muscle weakness. It should not be used to treat myofascial pain unless nothing else works.

SPASMS AND CRAMPS

Involuntary local muscle contraction is called a spasm. Many spasms are part of a self-perpetuating cycle, driven by pain. For example, long-standing myofascial pain may cause the development of spasm. Muscle injuries sustained in sports, for example, are often painful and may become spasmodic. Similarly, the pain from a broken bone or a herniated disk pressing on a nerve may cause spasm of the muscles around the bone or supplied by the pinched, painful nerve.

When an injury or disease sends pain impulses to the brain, the brain may return a message that increases the degree of contraction of muscles in and around the painful area. This increased contraction is spasm. It could be considered your body's attempt to keep a painful area from moving too much—tightening the muscles to act like a cast or splint.

All spasms interfere with normal muscle movement and are painful to varying degrees. The muscle spasm in the low back associated with a herniated disk may be as painful as the pain from the pinched nerve itself. The pain in the muscle spasm comes from the irritation of nerves within the tightened muscle, which is caused by chemicals produced by the spasm itself.

The intense muscle contraction of a spasm requires excessive muscle work, which requires a lot more fuel than usual. However, this excessive need is not met. The blood supply to an area of spasm is inadequate to feed the hungry, overworked muscle. As a result of this "unsatisfied hunger," the muscle generates acid. This acid and other by-products of the spasm irritate nerves within the muscle. These nerves send pain messages to the brain, which in turn sends back messages furthering the spasm and the pain. This leads to a downward spiral of progressively more pain and spasm.

Spasms are diagnosed by touching the muscle in question and discerning excessive tightness. However, spasm cannot be seen on an X ray and may not be detectable by any so-called objective tests.

Cramps are another type of muscle reaction to overuse and not necessarily associated with myofascial pain or trigger points. Muscle cramps, the kind we all have had at one point or other, are a type of severe short-lived spasm involving a whole muscle or group of muscles. Cramps can occur after exposure to cold or repetitive or prolonged muscle contraction from exercise. Remember the cramps you felt in your calves or other leg muscles while swimming in very cold water off the coast of Maine (or northern California or the Great Lakes) in the summertime? They came on suddenly, were severe, involved large parts of a muscle equally (a charley horse in the calf), and resolved slowly once you got out of the water and rubbed out the cramp. After the cramp subsided, residual local soreness may have existed for a few hours, if the cramp had been severe enough. A marathon runner may experience the same phenomenon as the swimmer, especially if he or she doesn't cool down. Writers and typists often experience cramps in their hands and arms from overuse.

Treatment of Spasms and Cramps

Spasmodic muscles have been treated successfully with massage, TENS, ultrasound stimulation, local heat or ice packs, various types of injections, and muscle relaxants. These treatments can relax the muscle, reducing its need for food; bring blood to the area to flush out the irritating acid; and break the spasm–pain cycle, usually with long-standing, and possibly permanent, relief.

When Painful Muscles Signal a Deeper Problem

The existence of myofascial pain or muscle spasm may be a signal that something more serious, or at least more complicated, underlies that pain. The muscle pain should not be treated without consideration of the cause of the painful condition. Poor lifestyle habits, overuse, painful facets, a herniated disk, and a malignant tumor eating at the spine can all cause myofascial pain and spasm. Treating the muscle pain without correcting its cause will not be successful and could be disastrous in the long run.

Some rehabilitation doctors often give short-term symptomatic relief—with physical therapies of various kinds—for myofascial pain or spasm without truly appreciating the cause of the problem. This is a particularly difficult issue when the cause of myofascial pain is another test-negative problem, such as painful facets or a degenerated but not herniated disk. If the facets or disks are not made less painful, the overlying muscle pain may often recur.

With treatment of the underlying pain "generator," the overlying myofascial pain or spasm will usually resolve either spontaneously or with a short course of physical therapy, accompanied by injections and the like if needed. Yet myofascial pain (not muscle spasm) may persist following successful surgery for a herniated disk or stenosis, which had caused severe sciatica. Sometimes a brief treatment for myofascial pain is needed even though the underlying cause of the original pain has been corrected. Some patients have adopted subtle postural changes to cope with their pain before surgery—for example, changes involving the muscles of the buttocks and pelvis that had caused a mild preoperative limp. These postural changes may have caused overuse or inappropriate use of various muscle groups that in turn caused myofascial pain, independent of the underlying pain from the pinched nerve. Following surgery, some patients may need some reha-bilitative help in ridding themselves of these learned but no longer use-ful postural changes to recondition their muscles.

Many athletes, exercise enthusiasts, and ballet dancers have chronic myofascial pain that is the result of overuse. They know it and cope with it, getting periodic treatment and modifying their training as needed. If different pain occurs in various areas of the body at different times, it is probably due to muscle strain. But if you have a particular area of strong persistent pain, see a doctor and have the pain evaluated.

Myofascial pain or muscle spasm, whether mild or severe, can be due to something serious or something benign. The man who rakes leaves for the first time in years and then, due to an excruciating back-ache, is confined to bed for three days has an overuse syndrome that will go away. Overuse gave him severe spasm. Even though it is inca-pacitating, it is not serious. The severity of his pain alone doesn't in-dicate a serious underlying disease.

THE ENIGMA OF FIBROMYALGIA

Fibromyalgia is a condition that involves widespread, chronic pain, lasting at least three months. The syndrome of fibromyalgia includes muscle pain and tenderness, with several points particularly tender to the touch spread over both sides of the body, above and below the waist. These points are generally both in the limbs and in the neck, thoracic area, or lower back.

Fatigue, depression, insomnia, migraine headaches, irritable bowel, and morning stiffness may all coexist with the pain. It is not clear if fibromyalgia is one disease or a collection of overlapping painful conditions. Like myofascial pain, this disease has no associated abnormalities noted on laboratory tests—it is another test-negative chronic painful condition.

Although fibromyalgia is still poorly understood, it is recognized more readily today than ten years ago. It is a widespread condition, seen in at least 10 percent of patients in general medical practice and 20 percent of patients in rheumatology clinics (rheumatologists, or arthritis doctors, often treat patients with this disease). Women are seven times more likely to be affected than men. Fibromyalgia is most common in people in their seventies, but it initially occurs between the ages of twenty and sixty. However, we don't know why people get this painful condition.

Patients with fibromyalgia are more likely to suffer from other chronic painful disorders such as female urethral syndrome, which resembles a bladder infection, the colicky pain of irritable bowel disease, and restless-leg syndrome. Normal nonpainful messages telling our brain mundane facts about our external environment or inside our bodies may be perceived as painful to patients with fibromyalgia or any of the above commonly related conditions.

Exciting research suggests that patients with fibromyalgia have an abnormally sensitized central nervous system (see chapter 1). Also, sensitization following trauma may be the cause of prolonged pain seen in some patients. For example, it may follow breast surgery or whiplash. There are increased rates of fibromyalgia following cervical spine injury, according to one study.

Certain diseases may also make us vulnerable for fibromyalgia. For example, 20 to 35 percent of patients with rheumatoid arthritis or lupus (another inflammatory condition) also suffer from fibromyalgia. It is also commonly seen in people with chronic low-back pain and common wear-and-tear arthritis. Inflammation or chronic pain and stress from these conditions may trigger or maintain an abnormal response to otherwise nonpainful sensations.

Of course, this begs the question, What about the 65 to 80 percent of patients with these conditions who don't have fibromyalgia? Possibly there is a genetic predisposition to fibromyalgia, which may be set off with the right (or wrong) conditions during life. In support of this, fibromyalgia is seen exceptionally commonly in female relatives of patients with fibromyalgia.

Treatment of Fibromyalgia

Medical treatments include muscle relaxants, low doses of tricyclic antidepressants, sleeping pills and sedatives, nonsteroidals, and trigger-point injections. Narcotics should be tried in treating moderate to severe chronic pain that doesn't respond to other medications.

Additionally, massage, stretching, biofeedback, relaxation exercises, and stress-reducing ergonomic furniture all may help fibromyalgia. Support groups may be beneficial as well. Clearly more research needs to be undertaken on fibromyalgia and related disorders.

OSTEOARTHRITIS: WEAR AND TEAR ON THE JOINTS

Arthritis is one of the most common health problems in the United States. Approximately forty-three million people, or one in six Americans, experience it, and two out of three sufferers are women. The most common form is degenerative arthritis, or osteoarthritis, which is characterized by chronic pain and stiffness around one or more joints. Wear and tear on the joints causes the cartilage covering the ends of the bone to deteriorate. Weight-bearing joints such as hips and knees are the most seriously affected. The shoulder joint can wear out as well because it gets such heavy use.

If you were athletic in your youth—pitching and hurling balls and other objects—you are at risk for serious arthritic shoulder problems. Skiers and runners can be subject to severe knee problems, even at relatively early ages. Being obese, however, may be as bad as, or even worse than, excessive exercise. Paradoxically, lack of use of joints—our unnaturally sedentary existence—may also contribute to arthritis. Sitting certainly isn't good for our backs. Genetics also appears to play a role in the development of arthritis.

Treating Painful Joints with Drugs

Arthritic joints contain a large quantity of corrosive chemicals produced by the body. These chemicals may be produced in response to joint trauma. They cause the breakdown of the soft cushion between the bones—the cartilage. This cushion also has a lubricating effect, facilitating smooth joint movement. The breakdown of joints in arthritis results in production of certain bodily substances—prostaglandins, among others—that irritate the membranes between the joints and the covering of the bones underlying the joints. All of these structures contain a rich supply of pain receptors.

Nonsteroidals (NSAIDs) reduce joint pain and stiffness by blocking production of prostaglandins. Note that many arthritic patients are undertreated for pain because the NSAIDs and Tylenol just aren't strong enough. The toxicities of NSAIDs and the deaths associated with their use are discussed in chapter 3. It might make more sense to use stronger and probably safer pain-relieving drugs, like well-prescribed narcotics, for controlling most moderate to severe pain not well controlled with NSAIDs, including that due to arthritis.

Glucosamine, a new and totally different type of substance from the drugs above, definitely helps reduce pain in many patients with arthritis for at least eight weeks. (The drug needs to be evaluated with long-term studies.) This drug has compared well with pain relievers like the NSAIDs. It is reputed to enhance growth of cartilage and is nontoxic to boot. However, I am far from convinced of its benefit in the long run. I have not found it helpful for patients with severe arthritis.

Hyalen and Synvisc are preparations of a drug (sodium hyaluronate) that was invented to "rejuvenate" the lost cartilage in deteriorated joints. The drug, which is usually injected into the knee on several occasions, relieves pain for up to six months and is supposed to restore the shock-absorbing qualities of the deteriorated joint. The injections may be repeated. We'll see what happens with this drug over the next few years. It is not a substitute for joint replacement if the joint is sufficiently deteriorated, but it may forestall the need for a joint replacement if used early enough in the degenerative process.

Joint Replacement

Wait as long as possible to replace any joints and be wary of a surgeon who encourages early joint replacement. These replacements for nature aren't perfect. They wear out within ten years or so—sometimes sooner and sometimes later, depending on the joint in question and the person wearing the joint. A heavy person may wear out a lower-extremity joint faster than a thinner person. Worn-out replacement joints also have to be replaced.

Artificial joints require a good round of rehabilitation before they work well. And guess who does the painful work or rehabilitation in spite of any pain medication you may take. If you do need a new joint, remember, use a surgeon with an excellent track record—one who has a lot of experience replacing the type of joint you need. A well-performed joint replacement, followed by excellent rehabilitation, can give you a new lease on life.

Rheumatoid Arthritis: The Body at War with Itself

Rheumatoid arthritis, fortunately, is more rare than osteoarthritis, affecting only about three million Americans, with women outnumbering men by two to three times. It is potentially more devastating than osteoarthritis and can affect people at any age—even children. It most commonly occurs between the ages of twenty and fifty.

Rheumatoid disease is a disorder in which your own immune system turns against you, inflaming and eventually chewing up your joints and anything around them—cartilage, tendon, and even bone—and inflaming your blood vessels as well, as if you yourself were a lethal bacterium or virus. Your own body declares war on you.

Rheumatoid arthritis usually attacks different joints than osteoarthritis, initially causing pain and stiffness. Eventually it may result in deformity of the knuckles. However, it can affect many other joints as well. It may make life a moment-to-moment hell, with devil's pitchforks jabbed into any joint attempting to move and even some completely at rest.

The disease may stop, seemingly as out of the blue as it started. It may slow down its rate of destruction. Or it may continue to progress, slowly crippling its victim.

Controlling the Disease to Control the Pain

Controlling the disease itself is of paramount importance because pain in severe rheumatoid arthritis is a reflection of the progression of the disease. Rheumatologists treat this disease by attempting to control the process and pain of inflammation with—you guessed it—massive doses of anti-inflammatory drugs, among other things. They also use drugs that pummel your own berserk immune system into submission. Various types of drugs used in treatment include:

- corticosteroids to reduce inflammation and diminish immunity

- methotrexate and Imuran (azothiaprine), anticancer drugs

- Plaquenil (hydroxychloroquine), a drug to control malaria

- Embrel (etanercept), a novel blocker of a chemical we all make as part of the natural inflammatory and immune processes

Using many of these drugs, alone or in combination, is like shooting rabbits with cannonballs. Yes, you'll kill the rabbits, but you'll destroy the garden along with them. Wouldn't it be better to use a selective device only for rabbits, preferably to trap the little garden destroyers?

Embrel blocks the action of tumor necrosis factor—an interesting name for a chemical that may *activate* our immune system in inflammation—and possibly help defend against cancer. This kind of drug is particularly promising because it, or its descendants, may control inflammation more specifically and with fewer side effects than some of the other drugs mentioned. The anti-immunological onslaught brought on by Embrel doesn't always arrest or slow down the disease, but often it does.

Unfortunately, staying on these immunological poisons for prolonged periods isn't exactly good for you. However, the goal is to make your condition improve with as little suffering as possible from the side effects of the treatment. That is often accomplished. With the development of more sophisticated, selective drugs, this disease may soon be treated more safely and effectively, limiting the pain, disfigurement, and sundry medical disabilities it causes. At the same time the treatment-related side effects will hopefully become minimal.

Treatment of the Pain with Drugs

Think of the women in tears with stiff, aching hands in the morning. In treating the pain of rheumatoid arthritis, some rheumatologists may rely too much on NSAIDs alone. Narcotics should be used to treat most moderate to severe pain. Combining NSAIDs with narcotics may allow the patient to take less of each, which entails fewer side effects.

OSTEOPOROSIS: THE PAIN OF DISINTEGRATING BONES

Osteoporosis is a serious public-health threat to more than twenty-eight million Americans, of whom 80 percent are women, according to the National Institutes of Health. Women aged fifty and over have a 40 percent risk of fracture over their lifetimes. It is a natural consequence of aging, although it is more common in women and Caucasians.

In spite of their appearance, bones are dynamic, constantly being broken down and remade. Their strength is due to the deposition of minerals within them. Osteoporosis (also osteopenia) results when the breakdown exceeds the buildup in bones, resulting in a net loss of their mineral content, making them fragile.

Bones naturally lose their minerals with age, but this loss is more serious in women after menopause, when the female body stops producing estrogen, a hormone that helps maintain bone mass. Other causes are diets low in calcium, which builds bones, hormonal disorders, prolonged treatment with corticosteroid drugs, alcoholism, smoking, a sedentary lifestyle, and a family history of osteoporosis.

In most cases, the first sign of serious osteoporosis is a fractured vertebra in the midspine. Wrists and hips are other prime candidates for fracture. The simplest everyday action may bring this on. A woman bends over to pick up a piece of paper from the floor and, arising from a stooped posture, experiences the sudden onset of paralyzing back pain. Amid grimaces, fear, and screams, she is taken to a hospital. X rays reveal the usual demineralized bones, at least one of which is collapsed, explaining the pain. She is admitted and put to bed and, if she is lucky, given enough around-the-clock narcotics to be comfortable. If she is not so analgesically blessed, she is given NSAIDs and some minor pain relievers on an insufficient basis, and suffers terribly. Some physicians try placing a brace on the patient, which may help a bit but often just makes the patient uncomfortable. Usually, within a few days, the pain may begin to subside, but the healing process may take up to two months.

Every time I see a menopausal patient or one who has had her ovaries removed, I ask her if she has had a bone-density test, a radiological evaluation of the degree of osteoporosis, at a facility where it is performed well.

A male veterinarian friend told me he went to his doctor with a cough that didn't go away. Concerned about pneumonia, the doctor got a chest X ray. The physician came back to his patient with two pieces of news. First, my friend didn't have pneumonia. He only had a nasty bronchitis. However, he did have an extraordinary case of osteoporosis, of which he was totally unaware. Unfortunately, all the research on the treatment of this disease has been done in women. So doctors are giving men the same drugs women use to control their disease, except for estrogen, of course. That strategy may undergo refinement as we learn more about male osteoporosis.

The specialists who treat osteoporosis advise which calcium supplements and medicines are the most effective. Nonprescription vitamins and minerals, such as vitamin D and calcium, *usually* are not enough. All of you naturalists who hate taking chemicals, please remember that. Various medications must be added to over-the-counter products to help restore bone density. Estrogen replacement in women is a first-line treatment.

However, many women with a history of breast or uterine cancer, or at risk for these diseases, cannot take estrogen—it could stimulate the growth of the cancer. Evista (raloxifene hydrochloride), a newer drug that binds to estrogen receptors while not stimulating the uterus or breasts as estrogen would, may help combat osteoporosis in those who cannot or should not take estrogen. It reduces bone breakdown and slows down the whole process of bone turnover. A thirty-six-month study of 7,705 postmenopausal osteoporotic women aged thirty-one to eighty showed that treatment with Evista increased bone-mineral density in the spine and hips and reduced the risk of vertebral fracture by 30 to 50 percent, compared with a group treated with an inactive substance. Other available drugs that inhibit the loss of bone are salmon calcitonin (Calcimar or Myacalcin—a nasal spray made from salmon eggs), and for somewhat more advanced cases, Fosomax (alendronate). Aridea (pamidronate) may also be used but must be given by periodic intravenous infusion.

Women and men should be evaluated if they seem to be at risk of developing osteoporosis because of taking medications like corticosteroids or, in women, because of hormone changes brought on by menopause or removal of the ovaries. Weight-bearing exercises like walking, bike riding, and weight lifting lessen the risk, especially when combined with exercises in which you bend backward. Crunches—bending forward—are not weight-bearing and actually increase the risk for lumbar compression fractures.

Severe osteoporosis is preventable and treatable, thanks in part to new medications that can strengthen bones. Rheumatologists and endocrinologists are the best ones to treat this disease. Unfortunately, once a woman—or, rarely, a man—with osteoporosis has a painful compression fracture, strengthening their bones is the least of their concerns. They want their pain controlled right then and there. And it should be.

If the pain from an osteoporotic compression fracture doesn't improve over two weeks, or cannot be controlled with narcotics and other medication due to significant side effects, vertebroplasty may be considered.

Treatment with Vertebroplasty

In brief, vertebroplasty is a procedure in which liquefied bone cement is injected through a needle into the collapsed bone. The liquid hardens in a matter of minutes to hours and stabilizes the bone. This keeps the bone from further collapse and almost miraculously, in about 90 percent of cases, gets rid of the pain. The procedure normally is carried out under intravenous anesthesia, using a CAT scanner or a specialized X-ray machine. The X-ray devices used to guide the procedure help the doctor monitor the placement of a needle into the weakened bone and the injection of the cement. There is an approximately 5 percent risk that the cement will leak out of the bone as it is injected, causing potentially serious complications by pressing on the nerves in or around the spine or traveling to blood vessels in the lungs. Most leaks, to date, have had little serious long-term consequences and required no treatment.

I love the dramatic gratification of helping patients through procedures like vertebroplasty. I learned how to perform the procedure in France in 1994 from the two groups of physicians who developed it— one in Amiens and one in Lyons. However, I see no need for vertebroplasty to be used for osteoporotic fractures if women, and in some cases men, have their bone density evaluated and treated early, before a compressive tragedy strikes.

In my experience, this procedure is appropriate in 15 percent or fewer of patients with osteoporosis. Most patients normally get better over time and just need pain medicine while they do so. Unfortunately, vertebroplasty appears to be overused in the United States today, sometimes by inexperienced physicians. If a patient can live on narcotic and nonnarcotic pain relievers, with few side effects, then he or she doesn't need vertebroplasty. Also, performing the procedure on a bone that collapsed more than three months earlier is usually unnecessary and will not relieve pain. Compression fractures normally heal within two months and spinal pain following that period is usually a result of the alteration of the spinal anatomy by the fracture. Increased pressure is placed on the facets attached to the vertebral bodies, or bones of the spine, involved in the fracture. The facets in, and even around, a fracture often become chronically painful and should be treated with pain medication or radiofrequency lesions (see chapter 6), not vertebroplasty.

Compression fractures usually occur in the elderly and, fortunately, Medicare recently agreed to cover vertebroplasty to treat these fractures. Private insurers traditionally cover procedures reimbursed by Medicare. It is unfortunate that medicine took many years to approve this valuable treatment, calling it experimental, in spite of the fact that it had been successfully and safely used since 1987. The track record of vertebroplasty has been documented in various articles in the medical literature analyzing the effects of this procedure in more than two hundred patients.

The Rabbi and the Devil's Trident

One of my elderly male patients, a famous rabbi, survived gastric cancer only to suffer severe back pain that was insufficiently controlled after several weeks with high doses of narcotics and other medication. His X rays and scans showed both osteoporosis and significant spinal arthritis—and, fortunately, no recurrent cancer. However, his scans showed several osteoporotic compression fractures, one of which appeared to be the devil's trident causing his exquisite pain. I recommended vertebroplasty to strengthen the vertebral body that caused his most severe back pain.

Being exceedingly conservative, he refused to undergo any procedure that involved any degree of risk, even the minimal risk of vertebroplasty. I tried to control his pain as best as I could with medication. He was also on medication to prevent further bone-mineral loss, but understood that this would not be terribly helpful for several years.

The rabbi came back three months later because his pain was worse than ever. I didn't understand why he hadn't healed. However, new scans showed that one of the vertebral bodies that had caused the original pain had collapsed more. Now it was pressing on a nerve root that travels under the lowest rib on the right. This gave him not only severe back pain but also burning, aching lower-abdominal pain.

Now he asked me to perform a vertebroplasty. But now I knew it wouldn't work. New scans revealed his bone was crushed in such a way that the cement would leak out onto his spinal cord or over the crushed nerve root. Also, a vertebroplasty would not take the pressure of the collapsed vertebral body off the nerve root. What the rabbi needed was surgery to drill the bone away from the root. He agreed to the surgery, and during the operation, it was obvious to my surgical colleague and me that the compressed nerve was crushed so badly that it might still cause pain even without the bone pressing on it. It was decided to cut the nerve in such a way as to relieve pain coming from it. At the same time, we sent a piece of the bone to the pathology laboratory to make sure the bone didn't have recurrent cancer that was causing ongoing collapse. During the operation we also injected bone cement into the collapsed bone, with the expectation of preventing it from collapsing further. It worked.

Within a few weeks, the rabbi was back to going to daily religious services and teaching—the joy of his life. We were all thrilled. I will always wonder whether, if he had had the vertebroplasty when he first saw me, he could have avoided the more complicated operation. I'll never know, and even now I am not sure he did the wrong thing by waiting. As I noted above, these fractures usually heal on their own over a few weeks.

KEY POINTS
About Musculoskeletal Pain

- For any persistent pain (over a month), don't allow any doctor to tell you "it's nothing" without making sure—with appropriate high-quality tests like an MRI.

- Persistent pain may signal an ongoing underlying cause. For example, if you have a tumor on your spine, then the back muscles may go into long-term spasm.

- Myofascial pain or a spasm can be a reaction to your lifestyle or reflect a serious underlying process.

- A plea to all women who are postmenopausal, have had their ovaries removed, or frequently have long periods of not menstruating: please see an osteoporosis specialist soon, obtain a high-quality bone-density test, and, if needed, get appropriate treatment to reverse the bone-weakening process of osteoporosis. Similarly, any men who are diagnosed with bone-mineral loss should be thoroughly evaluated and treated on a timely basis.

6

Your Aching Back: Pain from Head to Toe

Great blunders are often made, like large ropes, through a multitude of fibers.

—VICTOR HUGO

Your spine moves like a semirigid gooseneck lamp, with the greatest movement in your neck—which might move three hundred times a day—and your lower back. Whether you run a marathon or pick up a book from the floor, the disks lying between the bones (vertebrae) of your spine absorb the shocks of pressure and cushion the bones of your back to protect you from injury and pain. The wear and tear to these bones, disks, and related structures as we age is at the root of most back pain. Bones get arthritic, disks shrink or press on a nerve, supporting ligaments calcify, and so on.

There are thirty-two or thirty-three vertebrae in your spine. The seven top vertebrae, which support the skull and neck, are called the cervical spine and numbered C1 to C7. The next twelve vertebrae, which go down the back of the chest and connect to the ribs, are the thoracic spine (T1 to T12). The next five compose the lumbar spine (L1 to L5). Finally, the sacrum consists of five fused vertebrae, and the coccyx, or tailbone, is three or four fused vertebrae, at the bottom of the spine.

Each vertebra has a solid oval part in the front and a hollow arch

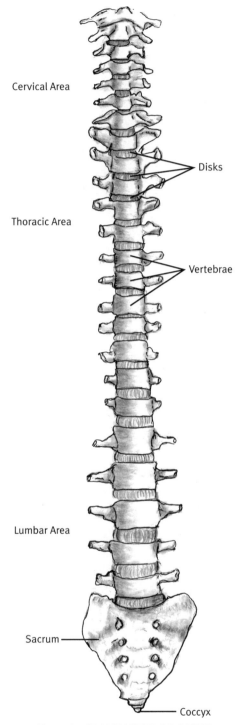

Cervical Area

Disks

Thoracic Area

Vertebrae

Lumbar Area

Sacrum

Coccyx

Figure 6   FRONT VIEW OF SPINE

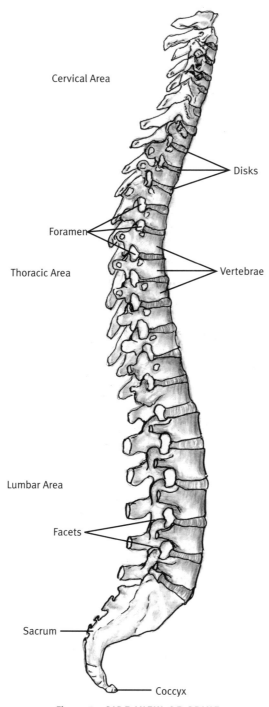

Cervical Area

Disks

Foramen

Thoracic Area

Vertebrae

Lumbar Area

Facets

Sacrum

Coccyx

Figure 7   SIDE VIEW OF SPINE

pointing toward the back. The sides of the arch are called lamina. A system of interlocking small joints called facets, located on the side of each vertebra, prevents us from turning too far and looking like the girl in *The Exorcist* who could spin her head all the way around. A U-shaped layer of thick yellow ligaments, just inside the arch and facets, further stabilizes the spine. The muscles of the back are attached to the back of the spine and, by pulling on these bones, stabilize and move the spine.

The vertebrae and interspersed disks support the weight of your spine. Within the vertebrae, under the arch and underlying ligaments, there is the spinal canal. In this protective, bony canal lies the delicate spinal cord, a cable of nerves about the thickness of your finger, and the nerves going into and out of the cord. The nerves within the cord carry messages up and down its length, to and from the brain, linking the brain with the peripheral nerves. There are sixty-two nerve roots that come off the side of the cord in pairs, thirty-one on the right and thirty-one on the left. A little hole, called a foramen, on either side of each vertebra, allows the nerve roots to exit the spinal canal. One pair exits at the level of each vertebra. Just below the place where the ribs reach the spine, the spinal cord ends and gives off a collection of nerve roots, called the cauda equina ("horse's tail" in Latin), that control feeling and movement from the groin down, as well as bowel, bladder, and sexual function.

The brain, spinal cord, cauda equina, and roots within the canal and foramen are wrapped in protective covering. Closest to the nervous tissue is an ultrathin membrane surrounded by colorless waterlike spinal fluid, which is contained by another thin membrane, the arachnoid, which looks like a spiderweb. A thick protective outer layer, the dura, completes the wrap. In the spinal canal, the dura is surrounded by the fat and veins of the epidural space.

HOW WEAR AND TEAR CREATES PAIN

Painful spinal disorders occur, in order of descending frequency, in the lumbar, cervical, and thoracic spine. The twenty-three disks between the vertebrae play a major role in the gradual process of spinal degeneration, pain, and disability. These semiflexible shock absorbers resemble checker pieces, with a shoe-leather covering called the annulus. They are filled with a substance like hard rubber, called the nucleus. Disks contain a large percentage of water, and after you turn thirty, they begin to dry out and become brittle and flatten (figure 15). Degenerated disks may crack and fissure, a potential cause of intrinsic

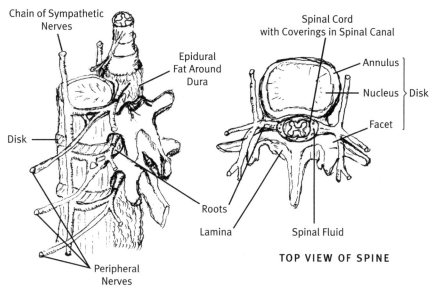

Chain of Sympathetic Nerves

Epidural Fat Around Dura

Disk

Roots

Lamina

Peripheral Nerves

**SIDE VIEW OF
CERVICAL OR THORACIC SPINE**

Spinal Cord with Coverings in Spinal Canal

Annulus

Nucleus } Disk

Facet

Spinal Fluid

TOP VIEW OF SPINE

Figure 8

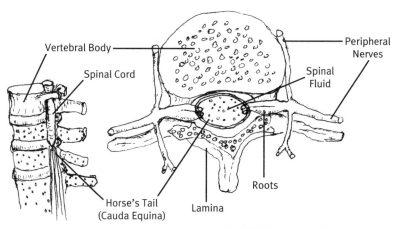

Vertebral Body

Spinal Cord

Peripheral Nerves

Spinal Fluid

Horse's Tail (Cauda Equina)

Lamina

Roots

**SIDE VIEW OF
LUMBAR SPINE**

TOP VIEW OF SPINE

Figure 9

disk-related, or discogenic, pain. More seriously, they may herniate (figures 10 to 14). The nucleus may ooze through a rip in the covering, causing pain or other neurological problems, especially if it presses on a sensitive nearby nerve root or the spinal cord.

Age and wear-and-tear-related loss of disk height also results in minor instability of the affected areas, with one vertebral body wiggling over another. To compensate for this instability, the supporting yellow ligaments thicken and compress the spinal canal and foramina. As we age, these bulging ligaments harden due to calcification and we develop pressure on the cord, the cauda equina, or the nerve roots exiting the spine. The narrowing process results in what we call stenosis, which can cause pain, weakness, or numbness. Sometimes the instability becomes serious and bones slip over one another significantly, causing narrowing of the spinal canal and foramina, which also results in stenosis. This instability can cause or worsen scoliosis.

If disks could be prevented from degenerating and losing height, or could be restored when they do degenerate, most spinal problems could be avoided. This is a serious challenge for preventive medicine and the biotechnology industry.

Facet Pain

As the spine loses height due to disk degeneration, the facets begin to carry undue weight. Remember, the facet is what keeps your head on straight. Facets are designed for creating stability more than bearing weight. Excess wear causes them to degenerate and some of them become arthritic and hurt—at times chronically. Anything that puts more weight on painful facets will cause further pain.

Facet pain may accompany osteoporosis, arthritis, or trauma such as whiplash. Painful facets can be identified by the pattern of referred pain, local tenderness overlying the facets, and pain elicited by certain body positions. Looking up while painting a ceiling or lying in sleep with the neck bent upward and backward often makes neck facet pain worse. Sitting or other activities that arch the back worsen lumbar or low-back facet pain. So a lumbar facet problem worsens during the day while the neck problem worsens at night. You go to bed with the back pain and may wake up with neck pain, depending on which one you have. (You may be unfortunate enough to have both, especially following a big whiplash injury in which you were thrown around, even with a seat belt.)

Thoracic facet pain may involve the thoracic spine anywhere from the shoulder blades down to the area over the lower ribs. Pain from thoracic facets usually doesn't travel to the side or front of the chest, unlike thoracic disk herniation, which compresses a nerve that travels under the ribs from the back to the front of the chest. Thoracic facet pain is usually worse during weight-bearing activities during the day, such as standing.

Discogenic Pain

Discogenic pain usually is described as deeper than facet pain. Disks are deeper than the facets and cannot be easily provoked by poking the area around the spine. Both facet pain and discogenic pain may be one-sided, but often they affect both sides. Facet and discogenic pain frequently coexist. Degenerated disks, noted on MRIs, may or may not be painful. However, painful disks are more likely to be degenerated and have a tear in the annulus than nonpainful disks. Ultimately, discography, mentioned later in this chapter, is the only way of determining whether a disk causes pain.

Unlike facet pain, lumbar discogenic pain may exist during the day and the night, the latter severe enough to impair sleep. Lumbar discogenic pain may be worsened by many activities—standing, walking, sitting, arising from a bent position, bending down, and even lying in bed, with the spine curving into the mattress. All of these activities may put vertical or bending-related stress on a degenerated painful disk, worsening symptoms.

Cervical discogenic pain may cause head, neck, shoulder, or arm pain.

True thoracic discogenic pain is rare. However, when it does occur, it is sometimes confused with other ailments like heart disease or reflux of the esophagus.

Herniated Disks

One of the more serious and common conditions of the degenerating spine is disk herniations, which can usually be diagnosed readily with a physical examination, guided by a good history, a high-quality MRI, and occasionally a CAT scan as well.

Most disk herniations occur at junctions where moving areas of the spine join relatively fixed areas. The neck and lower back—at or below the waist—produce the most problems. In the upper body, pain from a herniated disk squeezing a root in the neck frequently goes all the way down the arm. In the lumbar area, the most common sign of a herniated disk is pain going down one leg. A nerve root compressed by a herniated disk functions poorly, causing not only pain but also possible weakness, numbness, and loss of normal reflexes in the area

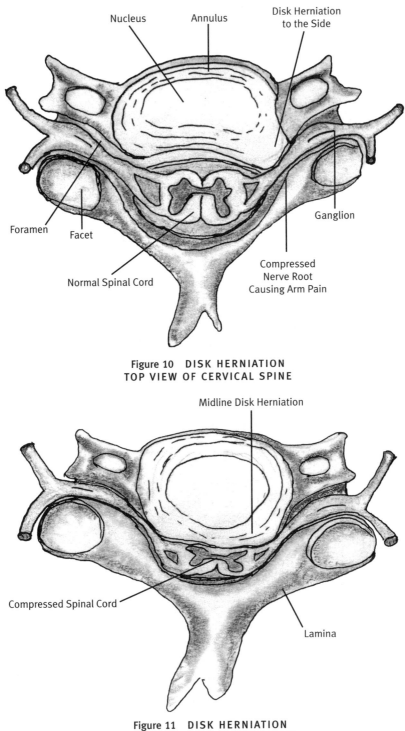

Nucleus   Annulus   Disk Herniation
to the Side

Foramen   Facet

Ganglion

Normal Spinal Cord

Compressed
Nerve Root
Causing Arm Pain

Figure 10 DISK HERNIATION
TOP VIEW OF CERVICAL SPINE

Midline Disk Herniation

Compressed Spinal Cord

Lamina

Figure 11 DISK HERNIATION
TOP VIEW OF CERVICAL SPINE

supplied by the root. (You won't kick properly when tapped with a re-flex hammer.)

The thoracic spine, behind the chest, is relatively safe from hernia-tion because it hardly moves. However, thoracic disk herniation does occur. Thoracic disk herniation brings varied symptoms such as band-like chest pain (the most common symptom), deep, dull pain behind the breastplate or stomach, pain between the shoulder blades, and oc-casionally tingling or weakness in the legs. Fortunately, in thoracic disk herniation, it is uncommon to see severe leg weakness or other symptoms suggesting an ill-functioning spinal cord, presumably squeezed by the herniated disk.

Cervical or thoracic herniated disks can compress the spinal cord. Similarly, large lumbar disks can compress the cauda equina signifi-cantly. These herniations affecting the cord or cauda can result in leg weakness, numbness, and bowel and bladder disturbance. Significant cauda equina compression also usually causes severe pain in both legs. If these symptoms occur, get an emergency evaluation by a skilled neu-rologist or neurosurgeon, possibly followed by surgery.

LOW-BACK PAIN

The lower back has to support the weight of the entire body above it and frequently bends, straightens after bending, and rotates, as we bipeds deal with things below the reach of our hands, or to the side of us. The lower spine takes more of a beating than other parts of the spine.

One-Sided Lumbar Pain

Pain on one side of the lower back is often due to four painful struc-tures, all of which must be treated in order to achieve a good result. The lower lumbar facets, the sacroiliac joint, myofascial pain of the side of the buttock, and bursitis of the hip on the same side may all contribute to this type of pain, which is diagnosed by history and physical examination. For example, the facets hurt during the day, es-pecially when you sit or arch your back, and the sacroiliac joint and especially the muscles and bursa may hurt more at night, when you lie on them. On examination, we try to elicit pain by poking or moving the suspected painful areas and reproducing the pain.

I don't know why one-sided back pain is so complicated, but I have seen this problem over and over again, and it is not well recognized by some physicians. Possibly people with one-sided low-back pain walk

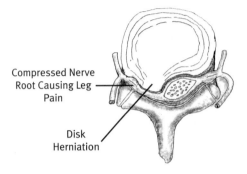

Compressed Nerve
Root Causing Leg
Pain

Disk
Herniation

Figure 12   TOP VIEW OF LUMBAR SPINE

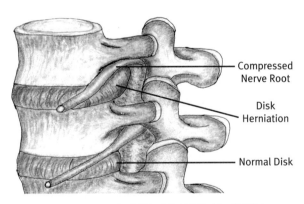

Compressed
Nerve Root

Disk
Herniation

Normal Disk

Figure 13   SIDE VIEW OF LUMBAR SPINE

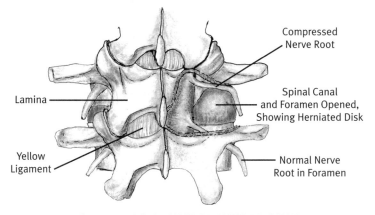

Compressed
Nerve Root

Lamina

Spinal Canal
and Foramen Opened,
Showing Herniated Disk

Yellow
Ligament

Normal Nerve
Root in Foramen

Figure 14   REAR VIEW OF LUMBAR SPINE

or hold themselves slightly crookedly, so more and more areas on one side become excessively worn or strained and painful. Did the facets hurt first and the sacroiliac joint, muscles, and hip bursa follow? Or vice versa? Is this the side on which the person always carries a heavy briefcase or purse? I usually treat this problem by a combination of medication injections, radiofrequency lesions of certain nerves, physical therapy, and some lifestyle changes.

Sciatica

True nerve-root pain, from pressure on or inflammation of a lower lumbar root, produces what is commonly referred to as sciatica, any pain coming down along the route of the sciatic nerve—from the low back to the buttock and down the leg to the foot. Pain that goes from the back down the leg below the knee can be due to compression of the lower nerve roots exiting the spine. It can also be caused by irritation of the sciatic nerve itself, a painful sacroiliac joint, myofascial pain of some buttock muscles, and occasionally from discogenic pain from a lower lumbar disk, for example. Lumbar facet pain usually doesn't travel down below the knee.

More seriously, sciatica can be caused by a lumbar disk herniation, stenosis, or tumor in the spine; compression of the nerves outside the spine from a disk or tumor; or, rarely, trauma to the sciatic nerve itself. I do not believe the sciatic nerve can be trapped by muscles in the buttock. Therefore, I would not advocate surgery to loosen purportedly tight muscles around the nerve. For most people, there is no significant benefit from such surgery.

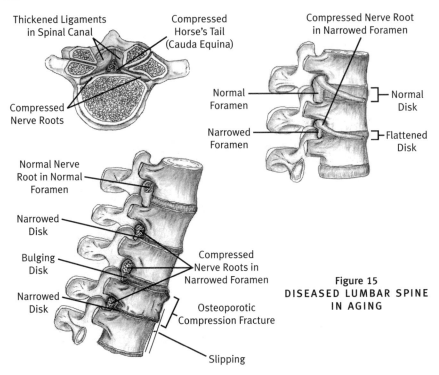

Figure 15
**DISEASED LUMBAR SPINE
IN AGING**

Lumbar Stenosis: Tightening of the Spinal Canal

Lumbar stenosis is a narrowing of the lower spinal canal that results in painful pressure on the nerves. Arthritis of the facets can cause it, as can the bulging and hardening of the yellow ligaments and disk degeneration. If back pain without leg pain is the major problem, and the pain gets worse when you sit or arch your back, some of the pain may be caused by arthritic facet joints.

This back pain may be treated by various means, including selectively destroying the nerves bringing pain impulses from the facets to the spinal cord, a safe, simple outpatient procedure.

If stenosis-related pain is severe, is exacerbated by exercise, or involves the legs (like sciatica), the solution becomes more complex. Walking increases heart rate, pumping more blood into the veins inside the already tight, stenotic spine. The veins dilate and press on nerves going into the legs, which in turn results in pain, weakness, or numbness. As soon as you sit, the heart function declines and the engorged veins shrink, easing the pressure on the nerves. You may experience pain even when standing still. This painful condition is called *neurogenic claudication*. Symptoms are similar to those of atherosclerosis, in which fatty deposits impair the blood supply and cause the legs to ache.

By studying the anatomy of your spine and possibly your blood vessels with MRIs, CAT scans, and other tests, physicians can usually identify the source of the problem. Many older people have a touch of both neurological and vascular problems. If the pulses in the feet, legs, and knees are good, the source is probably neurological and should show up on an MRI of the spine. When both neurological and vascular problems are present, deciding which condition to fix first depends on the specifics of the individual patient.

The pain of lumbar stenosis can be controlled for years with medication and modification of exercise, such as less walking. For those who do not wish to diminish their activity level, or if medication doesn't work, the best treatment for severe ongoing pain due to lumbar stenosis may be surgery, especially if leg weakness has developed. Physical therapy and purported pain-relieving epidural injections (discussed later in this chapter) are usually ineffective in patients with moderate to severe lumbar stenosis. Rehabilitation may be useful in some elderly patients following spinal surgery. The usual surgical treatment for this disease involves a laminectomy and facetectomy, discussed in detail later in this chapter.

Coccydynia: Painful Tailbone

Coccydynia, or painful coccyx, is not really low-back pain; rather it is usually due to some kind of trauma—like when you fall backward on the ice, landing on your buttocks and hitting the coccyx. It may resolve in a few days, but in a few cases it persists and becomes chronic. Then it is difficult to treat. Worse yet, it is often test-negative. On MRI, some people show evidence of a possible small, healed fracture by the time I see them, usually years after the fall.

A painful coccyx interferes with sitting, obviously, and therefore may be quite disabling. Sitting on a soft surface like a pillow helps. Some patients who came to me had used small pillows to ease the pain of prolonged sitting. Medication may help, but usually a medication regimen requires narcotics and possibly other types of pills.

Nerve blocks and epidurals are usually ineffective in the long run once coccydynia is chronic. Freezing or gently lesioning the nerves of the coccyx may help for several months. Partially destroying the ganglia of the nerves to the coccyx may be useful in some cases, but has a small risk of causing anal sphincter dysfunction. Surgically removing the coccyx almost never does anything except create new pain—possibly superimposed on the prior pain. Obviously, this suggests that some so-called coccydynia is often not even related to the coccyx at all!

THE DIAGNOSTIC CHALLENGE OF BACK PAIN

To properly diagnose painful spinal conditions, nothing less than excellent radiological studies are needed, because doctors must be able to see potentially painful anatomical abnormalities. To obtain the best studies, use a facility where an experienced neuroradiologist, who specializes in performing and interpreting studies on the nervous system, will supervise and interpret your radiological studies. If your insurance company won't pay for high-quality studies, you may need to challenge them or pay for them yourself. You wouldn't want your wedding photos taken with a disposable camera, so make sure you have the best pictures taken of your spine.

Plain X rays tell us little about the inside of the spine, but a flexion-extension X ray, taken while you bend your spine, can reveal possible slippage between vertebrae while you are in motion. To see what's going on inside your spine, you need an MRI or CAT scan—or both. MRIs provide images through the use of a magnetic field but do not use radiation. They are used to examine the spinal cord, nerves, roots, disks, and their coverings, and the spine itself. A CAT scan tells us if there are small fractures in the vertebrae that could lead to slippage. Small bony disk fragments or calcified ligaments are also best seen on a CAT scan.

MRIs and CAT scans are superseding myelograms, but this older test is still very useful. The technical and invasive nature of a myelogram makes it imperative that it be performed and interpreted by a neuroradiologist with significant experience. With a live "camera," radiological dye injected into the spinal fluid lets us see which nerves are compressed in different body positions. The myelogram is a powerful test that I still use routinely. This test often clinches diagnoses that have not been obtained by MRI or CAT scans. It is still the best radiological study for evaluating complex spinal problems.

Electromyography (EMG) is usually combined with a nerve conduction velocity (NCV). These tests measure the integrity of the spinal roots, peripheral nerves, and muscles. Diseased muscles or those supplied by damaged or dead nerve fibers behave differently electrically than those supplied by normal fibers. They are useful for diagnosing peripheral neuropathy or damaged peripheral nerves (see chapter 7). However, radiological tests clearly reveal the problem in most painful spinal conditions, rendering these electrical tests unnecessary 90 percent of the time.

Diagnostic nerve blocks and discography can help identify painful structures when nothing else can. Nerve blocks are used for diagnosis as well as treatment. Local anesthetics are injected around a nerve to block the transmission of pain impulses. Diagnostic nerve blocks should be used only to help confirm diagnoses suggested by other means. By themselves, blocks are not precise enough to pinpoint a source of pain. In the context of the total evaluation, these blocks may help identify the "pain generators."

The most important role of discography is in determining if a disk is painful. If an MRI reveals disk degeneration in one or several disks of a patient with poorly understood back or neck pain, a discogram may determine if a given disk (or disks) causes or contributes to the pain.

Evaluating Your Treatment Options

I specialize in procedures to relieve pain, yet I know that a painful spine should be given time, several weeks to a year, to heal on its own before surgery or other procedures are tried. In the meantime, pain can be controlled with medication and a severely restricted lifestyle for a few weeks to months as an acceptable alternative to pain-relieving surgery.

Weight loss, proper exercise, and lifestyle changes, as well as good pain medication, should be used intelligently and creatively to maximize your pain relief before you consider any surgery. If facet and discogenic pain do not improve with time, medication, and rest, they can usually be significantly relieved for years by simple surgical procedures outlined later.

Whether symptoms are due to sore facets, painful disks, or compressed roots from disk herniations or stenosis, exercise-related therapy should be avoided until symptoms begin to lessen considerably. At that point, physical therapy may be helpful in reconditioning someone who has been deprived of exercise for weeks.

Treating a Herniated Disk Without Surgery

Surgery definitely helps to resolve the symptoms of sciatica due to root compression from a herniated disk more quickly than conservative—

nonsurgical—treatment. However, if you are willing to wait it out and undergo nonsurgical treatment, it has been shown that ten years after the onset of sciatica, there is no difference in outcome between patients who had surgery and those who did not.

One study compared 166 sciatica patients who were treated with laminectomy (see page 125) with 417 others who were treated with only bed rest and a back brace. The study showed that 97 percent of the surgical patients had good results at one month compared with 76 percent of the bed-rest group. However, at six months, 99 percent of the group that had undergone the surgery reported good results, as did 93 percent of those who only rested in bed. I'm not suggesting you stay in bed for months or that you use a brace. But this study illustrates the value of deferring surgery if possible.

Why try to avoid surgery? Because spinal surgery always carries some small risk of infection, nerve damage, and even death. Also, once your spine has undergone surgery, even with good results, you may be more likely to suffer spinal problems later in life.

The amount of actual disk that is herniated, the severity of the pain and its associated neurological problems (weakness and numbness, compression of the delicate spinal cord), and the degree and length of disability all contribute to the decision for or against surgery. A herniated disk may rupture blood vessels and look enormous on an MRI. But the large disk herniation may in fact represent a moderate-sized disk fragment surrounded by a large blood clot or inflammatory cells, making a large mass. A good radiologist may be able to tell the difference between herniated disk and other material—a difference that may influence the decision for or against surgery.

Medications such as NSAIDs, narcotics, or drugs for neuropathic (nerve-related) pain may help. Go back to chapter 3 for more explanation on how these drugs can help relieve pain. A short course in oral steroids may also help. I give them for only two weeks.

Lifestyle changes can improve the quality of life following a disk herniation—and possibly save you from surgery. Lifting, coughing, and other forms of straining are bad for any herniated disk, as these activities make the disk bulge out more, further pressing on the root, worsening the pain, and increasing the possible need for surgery. Don't lift anything, including your baby or a purse weighing more than a pound. Take cough medicine if needed, use antihistamines if you sneeze due to allergies, and use stool softeners to avoid straining with bowel movements.

Local heat, massage, acupuncture, ultrasound, and TENS (see chapter 2) may all help reduce pain temporarily, while the herniated disk has a chance to shrink—which is how you get better. However, none of these therapies will heal the disk and permanently reduce the pain it created. The body actually "eats up" the disk herniation over time. In 80 percent of patients with lumbar and 70 percent of patients with cervical disk herniations who experience pain and other symptoms, conservative or nonsurgical therapy works. Remember that!

Either the herniated disk shrinks and you improve, or you continue to suffer, or you choose surgery. If symptoms have not begun to resolve after a month (that doesn't mean they have completely resolved), it may not be possible to wait longer before getting surgery. Again many factors have to be considered, including your personality, lifestyle, professional commitments, general health, and the nature and history of your spinal problems.

Low-back and leg pain due to disk herniations call for conservative treatment such as medication, rest as needed, and the other remedies described above. If you wish to use anything else, like a lumbar support for a while, do so for a few weeks if you think it makes you feel better. It isn't clear that these devices, or any others like them, really do anything to make you heal, except possibly reminding you not to bend too suddenly. If used for extensive periods, they weaken your back.

Disk herniations in the neck. Rest your neck and take pain medication. Sleep on your back to keep the nerves in the neck from being jabbed by disks or arthritic protuberances as you turn your head to the side. Use a strong sleeping pill with your pain medication if needed, as most adults can't sleep on their backs for a whole night.

Wearing a soft cervical collar will help you rest your neck. Use it for up to two weeks, day and night. Later, for several months and for intermittent pain flare-ups thereafter, this collar may be used to help you sleep at night—on your back, without turning your head. The collar should be fitted so it is comfortable yet supportive. The closure should be placed in the front, not the back—which is not what most physicians and the people selling these collars will say. To achieve the best relief of arm pain and other arm symptoms from a disk herniation, the collar should bend the head slightly forward, maximally opening the tight foramen and area around the root. This position is best reinforced by wearing the thick part of the collar behind the neck and the smaller part of the collar (where the closure is) in the front of the neck.

Epidural Steroid Injections

Epidural steroid injections can relieve pain from a relatively new disk herniation while it is given time to heal on its own. One of the reasons we have pain when nerve roots are pressed by a disk is that nerves under pressure become swollen and inflamed. They actually expand against whatever is already pressing on them, making the pressure worse and increasing the pain. Theoretically, steroids work by reducing swelling or inflammation within the nerve root, causing it to shrink, reducing the pressure on it and the pain impulses generated by the area under pressure. Besides acting on the swollen, inflamed nerves, the liquid in the epidural also flushes away the body chemicals produced by the disk herniation that cause root inflammation and more nerve-root pain.

Studies on epidurals show that they work well for a very small, specific group of people—those under forty, in pain less than three months, suffering from disk herniations and tears in the annulus, who have not had prior surgery. In fact, in most cases of sciatica due to disk herniations, epidurals do not relieve leg pain on a long-term basis or reduce the need for eventual surgery. Epidurals are not very effective in treating the pain from significant stenosis.

An epidural cannot be performed safely if you are taking a blood thinner, such as Coumadin, because it could result in massive bleeding within the spinal canal. A blood clot from this trauma could create pressure on the cauda equina or the spinal cord and cause permanent nerve damage. If a patient taking Coumadin to prevent strokes is taken off the medication the requisite several days prior to the injection, it raises the risk of stroke.

Accidental puncture of the dura and arachnoid encasing the spinal fluid is another risk of this procedure. The spinal fluid may leak into the epidural space. Normally, the hole in the system heals. When it doesn't, the fluid leaks whenever you sit or stand, causing severe headache. This condition requires treatment until the leak stops.

Epiduroscopy: A Look Inside Your Spine

Epiduroscopy, an increasingly used technique in which a fiber-optic scope is inserted into the epidural space to identify and treat epidural scars, is not a practical diagnostic or useful therapeutic tool in dealing with back pain. The same is true of passing catheters and injecting chemicals into the epidural space to relieve pain from scars. Epiduroscopy may show inflamed nerve roots in some patients with persistent pain following surgery, but then again so can less costly and noninvasive tests, such as high-quality MRIs.

Even proponents of these techniques admit that the treated pain, if it goes away at all, usually recurs within a few months or less. Scars in any postoperative site exist and will only re-form if an attempt is made to cut them. They are part of the healing process—a reaction to invasion of the body. Scars within nerves may cause pain and numbness or weakness, but cannot be successfully removed—they are an intrinsic part of nerve damage. The neuropathic pain due to such scars can be treated, however.

Facet and Nerve-Root Blocks

Local anesthetics alone or mixed with corticosteroids can be injected into the facets or over the nerves that carry sensation—including pain impulses—from the facets. These latter nerves are branches of larger nerves that supply the muscles and skin of the neck and back. Other targets for these injections are the nerve roots exiting the spine and other peripheral nerves. These injections are called facet, branch, root, or nerve blocks, respectively. Unlike epidurals, these blocks are primarily diagnostic tools, with possible therapeutic effects. Whatever therapeutic effect such injections may have usually diminishes with time.

These blocks usually do *not* work on a long-term basis. Moreover, it is impossible to predict who is likely to experience long-term benefit from nerve blocks. Repeated facet and nerve blocks are not an efficient, cost-effective means of controlling chronic pain. Unfortunately, these blocks are as overused by pain-management specialists as fusions are by spine surgeons, EMGs by neurologists, and excessive physical therapy by physiatrists.

Nerve and facet blocks must be performed by a skilled physician. Blocks involving spinal structures should be performed using high-quality X-ray guidance to safely and accurately place the needle and verify the placement of the injected liquids.

Cutting Off the Pain Impulse: Radiofrequency Lesioning

One method I use following a successful diagnosis with nerve blocks involves using radiofrequency energy to achieve highly selective, partial or total destruction of nerves carrying pain impulses. These nerves can be carrying pain from facets, disks, nerve roots, or areas of the body sending impulses up the peripheral nerves to specific nerve roots. The energy is delivered through a wire electrode placed into the body over a specific nerve or nerves. Such a destruction of nerves is called a lesion. The extent of intentional nerve damage depends on the nerve being lesioned. Certain nerves can tolerate more of a lesion than others without side effects. The trick is to know which nerves to damage, and by how much.

Eventually, the lesioned nerves may grow back and pain may recur. Fortunately, for most people, pain does not recur in the lesioned area. If necessary, you can be re-treated with radiofrequency lesioning, with excellent long-term results.

Radiofrequency lesioning is a highly effective, safe, proven treatment for chronic pain, providing years of relief. It is performed with radiological guidance, in an outpatient setting, using local or mild intravenous anesthesia. You can usually return to work later the same day, or certainly by the following day.

If you have not benefited from standard conservative therapy for spinal pain, certain radiofrequency procedures provide *at least* eighteen months of significant pain relief, meaning at least a 50 percent reduction, without using any more pain medication or changing your lifestyle. The goal of pain therapy is to restore function and diminish the need for medication.

Studies have shown neck, head, and facial pain coming from painful cervical spinal structures may be significantly improved in more than 80 percent of patients. Similarly, pain in the lower shoulders, between the shoulder blades, and in the spine behind the ribs may be significantly reduced in 90 percent of patients. Finally, low-back and related buttock, hip, groin, thigh, and upper-leg pain may be significantly reduced in at least 45 percent of patients. In my experience it is closer to 65 percent. These techniques have been applied to patients with spine-related pain from cancer, with good, lasting results.

In the area of discogenic pain, these minimally invasive techniques compete with major surgery—fusions. As you read this section—and a later one on fusions—you will note that, without question, I strongly oppose fusions for truly discogenic pain.

Intradiscal radiofrequency lesioning is a relatively new technique for treating discogenic pain. This takes an hour or two, depending on the location of the disk(s) being lesioned and the number of disks involved. It is performed similarly to other radiofrequency procedures. It may be used for discogenic pain in the low back and neck. The radiofrequency procedure is effective and you should feel relief quickly and resume your normal lifestyle within a few days.

The mechanism underlying the effectiveness of this procedure is not well understood. Degenerated disks have nerves that grow into the nucleus, along its cracks, from the annulus. It may be that this procedure destroys those nerves within the disk, preventing them from transmitting pain impulses to the brain.

IDET and Laser Treatment for Low-Back Pain

A similar, even newer procedure called IDET (intradiscal electrothermal lysis) uses conductive heat, like that emitted from a toaster, to treat disk-related pain. In this procedure, a toaster-wire-like device is threaded carefully into the offending disk(s), and the interior of the disk and overlying annulus is heated for about fifteen minutes, after which the wire is removed. It is theorized that this technique changes the chemical structure of the disk for the better, eventually making it stronger. With this improvement, pain subsides.

Lasers also have been used to treat painful disks, and this technique is the oldest. Laser treatment involves a small pencil-like object being inserted into the disk, similar to the radiofrequency electrode above, except that it is much larger. The nucleus of the disk is then treated with laser energy for a short period. The proponents of this technique contend that they are making a vacuum within the disk, so that the nucleus sucks in the outer parts of a weakened, protruding disk, making it less painful.

Both of these latter techniques may only be used in the lumbar spine, due to the size of the probes used. Cervical disks are much narrower than lumbar disks, and thoracic disks are difficult to enter safely with such thick probes. Both of these techniques must be performed with X-ray guidance. The recovery times after these procedures differ. The IDET procedure may take two to three months of recovery. In fact, the preexisting pain may increase transiently following the procedure. The laser procedure has a recovery period of a few days.

The outcome and the method of pain control from any of these procedures are not well established. Therefore, it is impossible to decide which, if any, is superior to the others. Claims about the last two procedures indicate that 75 percent of patients with one painful lumbar disk will achieve significant long-term benefit. At least 70 percent of the fifteen patients I have treated with the radiofrequency technique have had greater than 80 percent reduction in their pain. At this point, none of these claims are supported by well-designed academic studies.

Use of IDET seems to be sweeping the country, but it has not yet been evaluated in a rigorous manner. Well-designed studies must be conducted to determine the relative efficacy and limitations of all these techniques to control this common type of pain.

Cryoanalgesia

Cryoanalgesia uses cold instead of heat to create a smaller lesion; it is less destructive than traditional radiofrequency lesioning. Cryoanalgesia can be used safely on peripheral nerves. However, lesions made with this technique last only approximately three months and may have to be repeated. Aside from the short duration of effect, the cryoprobe, the device that must enter the body to make the lesion, is about as thick as a pencil, while a radiofrequency probe is as thin as a standard hypodermic needle. Therefore it is more difficult to use and really can't compete with the utility and efficacy of the radiofrequency technique for lesioning nerves around the spine.

The Woman with the Crooked Spine

Mariana Rideau is a patient who taught me more about referred pain from the spine than any textbook ever did. At the time I met her, she was fifty-eight and was referred to me by a neurological colleague for pain control. She is a prominent, highly active businesswoman who had suffered from scoliosis since adolescence. She had never been treated surgically and had not been incapacitated by back pain until the year before she came to see me. She is a strong woman who had survived breast cancer and was coping with chronic reflux esophagitis, which had required her to sleep sitting up in a chair for the preceding two years.

Mariana had pain in her entire spine and occasional severe right-sided headaches. Her thoraco-lumbar pain had become incapacitating. For most of us, being incapacitated is bad enough. However, she had two particular reasons for not wanting to become incapacitated. First, she had seen her mother become an invalid from rheumatoid arthritis while Mariana was still in school. She never wanted to end up like that. Second, she had been raised by her father to be a high-powered business executive, just as he was. She loved her work as much as, if not more than, just about anything else in her life. She wanted to continue to work at all costs. I didn't know what to do at first, but agreed to try to help her.

Her neurological exam was essentially normal. I started her on a mixed regimen of narcotics and Tylenol and evaluated her extensively radiologically, including with MRIs and a CAT/myelogram. She had significant scoliosis, and I felt this was responsible for most of her pain. I referred her to both a neurosurgical colleague and an eminent orthopedic scoliosis expert.

The neurosurgeon decided she did not have any surgical problem from his point of view. The orthopedist originally agreed to operate on her but later changed his mind, stating he felt she was not psychologically strong enough. Her films were sent to various other spine specialists and most agreed she was not a suitable candidate for scoliosis surgery. Mariana was devastated and asked me what I could do other than prescribing the same drugs she was already taking, which worked only moderately and somewhat impaired her alertness at key business-decision-making moments.

I decided to evaluate the potential pain generators in her spine with diagnostic blocks and, where appropriate, lesion them. Over a period of time, I eventually lesioned many of her thoracic facets, as well as some of her lumbar and cervical facets, essentially abolishing her thoracic, neck, and head pain and significantly reducing her lumbar pain. Her case taught me multiple new patterns of referred pain that I have since seen repeatedly in other patients with scoliosis and thoracic pain syndromes.

Mariana continues to lead an active life several years after I met her, working more than twelve hours daily as a business executive. Her crooked spine still hurts, but with some pain medication she is able to work according to her brutal schedule.

The Bond Trader's Sciatica

Franklin Jones, thirty-six, is a Wall Street bond trader. He had undergone lumbar disk surgery in January 1998 for the relief of left-leg "sciatica," with excellent results, until the spontaneous occurrence of excruciating low-back pain two weeks before he consulted me. His pain was so severe that he consulted his neurosurgeon, who, in consultation with the patient's neurologist, ordered an MRI, which revealed not compressed nerves but an annular tear associated with a moderate disk protrusion at the level above his surgical site. He had no leg pain and had a normal examination with the exception of significant low-back spasm. It was concluded that he didn't require a surgical procedure and that bed rest and oral medication should help him recover. Two weeks after the onset of his pain he was no better and had been disabled at home, unable to work. His pain disturbed his sleep and plagued him all day long, improving only partially when he was flat on his back.

Franklin had three small children to support and was concerned about his income and job future. He was referred to me and I concurred that his pain was probably due to the torn annulus, although his MRI suggested that the disk below, which had already been operated on, could also be a good candidate for causing pain. The MRI also suggested that his spine may have been unstable at the prior surgical level, another cause of pain that ultimately could lead to re-operation and fusion.

I ordered an X ray to determine whether his spine was in fact stable, changed his medication, and gave him an epidural steroid injection. The latter procedure was performed, against my better judgment, at his request, because he wanted to go back to work. I explained to him that if it worked I would eat his Borsalino hat at Lutece. The X rays demonstrated that his spine was stable. The epidural lasted two days, the medication helped only moderately and made him sleepy, he kept his hat, and I ate something far better at another restaurant.

We decided to investigate him with a discogram, which revealed that the disk with the annular tear was the cause of his pain. Ultimately he was treated with the radiofrequency disk/annulus heating procedure and within three days was back to work with no pain. Because of the weakened, protruding disk, he was cautioned to avoid lifting, bending, and turning of his lower spine, so as to avoid a full disk herniation, possibly requiring further surgery. At work, colleagues commented on how freely he moved, with no facial expression suggesting any discomfort. He required no medication and has done well in the two years since the procedure. Before writing this story, I checked on him. He rates his sustained improvement as 75 percent.

TREATING BACK PAIN WITH SURGERY

If you have significant pain, with or without weakness or significant numbness, due to disk herniation, significant spinal stenosis, or gross instability in the spine, you should proceed to surgery sooner rather than later. Conservative therapy doesn't work well in conditions where nerves are being severely compromised. Obviously, surgery is required if there is an ongoing disability or, in the neck and thoracic areas, the potential for permanent injury to the spinal cord.

In general, any disk in the neck or thoracic spine pressing on the spinal cord and causing dysfunction should be removed quickly. The greater the dysfunction and the more quickly it appeared, the greater the urgency of surgery to avoid irreversible damage.

Weakness of the muscles needed to raise the foot off the ground, or of those keeping your knee straight, is a particularly troublesome sign of a lumbar disk herniation. If this weakness doesn't resolve, you could end up with a permanent inability to walk normally. A herniated disk in the neck or thoracic area that causes arm or chest pain and is pressing on the spinal cord, causing symptoms of leg weakness, should be treated promptly with surgery. Bowel or bladder dysfunction attributable to pressure on the spinal cord or cauda equina is cause for rapid surgical removal of the source of pressure.

Even without weakness or other physical abnormalities, ongoing disabling pain attributable to a disk herniation that shows up clearly in quality radiological studies also may result in surgery if a reasonable course of conservative therapy is unsuccessful.

Spinal surgery means that the inside of your spine is being invaded and there is potential for serious side effects and complications. Yet, with the correct diagnosis and excellent surgical treatment, the majority of patients improve significantly following most types of spinal surgery. Most spinal surgery is performed to remove pressure from the spinal cord or roots, relieving pain or disability. The pressure is usually due to herniated disks or enlarged, calcified ligaments and deposits of arthritic bone. This kind of surgery involves gaining access to the spinal canal and foramen where the cord, cauda equina, and roots reside. Operations for treating lumbar disk herniations and stenosis are performed from the back. To widen either the spinal canal or the foramen, various structures are removed—all or part of the lamina surrounding the spinal canal (laminectomy or laminotomy), some of the underlying ligaments, and sometimes parts of the facet (facetectomy or foramenotomy).

A simple *lumbar discectomy* is the most common spinal surgical procedure. In this one-hour operation, the portion of disk that is herniated, pressing on the roots, is removed. Usually, within six weeks following surgery, you should be able to resume normal activity. Initial open lumbar disk surgery produces good to excellent results in about 90 percent of patients. Five years following surgery, most people are quite satisfied with their sustained pain relief. It is not at all clear that this good outcome is achieved by the newer discectomy techniques. These include microdiscectomy, which is performed through a smaller incision with the aid of an operating microscope, or percutaneous or endoscopic discectomy, performed by pushing specialized instruments through the skin without an incision.

Subsequent open discectomy at a previously operated site is less successful than initial surgery. Common reasons for failure following any disk surgery include inadequate removal of herniated disk material and preexisting or surgically related nerve damage. If shortly following surgery your leg pain is dramatically worse or you have more weakness or numbness than before, you may have sustained nerve damage during surgery.

Laminectomy, partial facetectomy, and *possible foramenotomy,* the usual procedures for treating lumbar stenosis, open a tight spinal canal and the foramen, relieving pressure on the roots. This is a good operation for the elderly with at least moderate stenosis and it should be pursued aggressively. Two weeks after the operation, you should feel better. Studies reveal a high level of success with up to 85 percent good to excellent relief of symptoms. When people don't respond well with this surgery, it is often because the surgeon failed to open sufficiently the sides of the spinal canal or the foramen, so the roots remain squeezed. A few patients have so many spinal problems that it is impossible to address all of them effectively through this procedure.

Because stenosis is usually a condition of diffusely aging spines, from 30 to 40 percent of those who have the operation do not get a long-lasting benefit. Disabling symptoms of stenosis can be corrected in one operation with excellent results. However, the aging process and spinal degeneration continue. Over several years, another spinal level may begin to cause problems, eventually requiring surgical treatment. Surgery is not a cure for the aging process, but for the pain of severe stenosis limiting the ability to walk, surgery can give gratifying results.

In the cervical and thoracic spine, *foramenotomy* is also performed from the back. Judicious use of this simple operation to relieve pressure on the roots from disk herniations or stenosis not involving the spinal canal or underlying cord may allow you to avoid a fusion, a much more complicated operation.

Spinal fusions can correct the deformity and side effects of scoliosis and they can reconstruct spines broken in accidents. They are also performed to correct spines that are unstable with one vertebra slipping over another, causing pain or dysfunction (figure 15). Also, cervical and thoracic disk herniations pressing on the spinal cord can be removed only by approaching the spine from the front of the body. This also requires a fusion. Fusions bond one or more spinal vertebrae together with another piece of bone (your own or from a bone bank) or metal hardware. The rate of failed fusion increases with the number of spinal levels fused.

Cervical fusion is the biggest category (48 percent), followed by lumbar fusion (33 percent) and thoracic (13 percent). Most cervical fusions are performed from the front of the neck. These operations are performed on a regular basis today with good results and require less than a week of hospital stay and a three-month recovery. Results are good to excellent in more than 87 percent of cases.

Sixteen to about 90 percent of patients reportedly benefit from lumbar fusions. This wide range of outcomes raises serious questions about who really needs this kind of surgery. At least 30 percent of those who undergo lumbar fusion have serious complications later, including severe pain. Lumbar fusion should not be done unless the vertebrae keep slipping back and forth, hitting the roots, causing disabling, poorly controlled leg pain, weakness, numbness, and bowel or bladder problems. Even if your back slips and causes pain, if you can find a way to live with it, do not have a fusion because the fusion itself can cause chronic pain. There are no data suggesting fusion is better than any other nonsurgical therapy or simpler surgery in treating pain from disk herniations or uncomplicated stenosis. Yet, 51 percent of lumbar fusions are performed for discogenic pain and 11 percent for stenosis.

Thoracic fusion can correct scoliosis, including lower thoracic–upper lumbar deformities due to cerebral palsy, polio, or other neurological diseases. This operation is also used to treat vertebrae damaged by accidents, infections, or tumors. Such fusions approach the spine through the back or the chest cavity, or both, and are clearly "big surgery" with a potentially long, painful recovery and should be undertaken only when necessary.

The United States is in the midst of an epidemic of spinal fusion not unlike other surgical fads of the past. From 1995 to 1996, neck and thoracic fusion each increased close to threefold and lumbar fusion by 21 percent. Our nation has the highest incidence of spinal surgery in the developed world, by far, and the rate of fusion varies according to region. More fusions are performed in the Midwest and South than in the Northeast, which does more than the West. This is not because an Alabama back differs from a Boston back, but because of the biases of physicians.

Any spinal fusion distorts the normal movement of your spine. The segments above and below the fused area move excessively, compensating for the lack of movement in the fused segment. The excessive movement accelerates wear. Disks herniate and stenosis occurs, problems that must be addressed over the five to ten years following fusion, often with more surgery, and possibly even further fusion. Fusions should be performed only if there is no other way to relieve the pain or dysfunction.

For those with significant pain and disability persisting more than two months following any spinal surgery, appropriate treatment requires a proper diagnosis. Causes of failed surgery include nerve damage; inadequate removal of structures pressing on the nerves; postoperative disk herniations, spinal slippage, and infection; or simply the wrong initial diagnosis and treatment.

KEY POINTS
About Back Pain

- Go to the doctor immediately if you have profound back pain and numbness or weakness.

- If back pain is moderate to severe, wait to see if it gets better before you go for a consultation.

- If you have pain and no numbness or weakness, take pain-relieving medicine such as Tylenol, NSAIDs, or even mild narcotics like codeine for five or ten days.

- Have a lumbar (low-back) fusion if you are experiencing ongoing slippage of the spine causing severe leg pain and possibly weakness and numbness.

- Back pain alone is usually not a good reason to have a fusion.

- There are other, less invasive procedures than fusion to correct chronic back problems, as well as medications to control pain.

- Both simple disk and stenosis surgery usually give gratifying results when performed for an appropriate anatomical problem by an experienced surgeon.

- Stenosis surgery is not a cure for the aging process.

- If you still have pain following spine surgery, get a proper diagnosis to see what else can be done before embarking on years or even a life of chronic pain and its management.

7

The Nerve of That Pain: Neuropathic Pain

As I was going up the stair
I met a man who was not there.
He wasn't there again today.
I wish, I wish he'd stay away.

—HUGHES MEARNS

Unlike the man who wasn't there, neuropathic pain definitely exists. But like the absent man, we're often not sure *why* it occurs at all, much less why it occurs *when* it does. It doesn't follow the rules of pain. It doesn't go away when you heal. Worse yet, the pain may come on spontaneously, unpredictably, for no apparent reason, at some times and not others. Or it may exist all the time, with spontaneous fluctuations in severity. Like the man in the poem, this pain is unfamiliar to us—it feels so *strange*. The skin involved in the painful area may be abnormally sensitive to the lightest touch or could even be numb and still be excruciatingly painful. Neuropathic pain is caused by painful stimulation of, damage to, or dysfunction of nerves in the peripheral or central nervous system.

Much commonly experienced neuropathic pain has a well-defined cause and can be effectively treated by eliminating the cause. A lumbar disk herniates and compresses a nerve root, causing shooting, burning pain or numbness in the leg. Remove the pressure of the disk and the pain usually goes away. However, when pain has no obvious stimulus it is far more difficult to treat. This type of pain is caused by the nervous system itself, which for some reason is not behaving normally. It may be the result of sensitization or other mechanisms that short-circuit the nervous system or increase excitability of peripheral nerves, spinal roots, and the neurons within the central nervous system's pain pathways.

An actual case history illustrates the tragedy of neuropathic pain and the frustration of doctors trying to treat it. Quentin Smith is forty and has been disabled for several years—since an automobile accident fractured his pelvis and damaged the nerves going into his right leg, with subsequent numbness, weakness, and searing pain in the leg. The pain has never been well controlled by his doctors and he has never been referred to a pain specialist. He began drinking in a vain attempt to relieve his pain.

In moments of desperation, Smith gets much of his pain care through the revolving-door clinics known as emergency rooms. He has become a regular in the emergency room of a medium-sized rural hospital. The nurses cringe when they see him because there is not much they can do for him. On one of his many visits he reports particularly severe burning and stabbing pain in his right leg.

"The pain never goes away," he says. "Sometimes I just can't stand it anymore." The doctors prescribe Demerol injections and a small supply of oral narcotics, which temporarily dull his pain. But the pain will recur and he will return to the ER, each time frustrated and angry and more difficult to pacify and treat.

People who suffer from neuropathic pain sometimes go from doctor to doctor seeking relief. They are often suspected of exaggerating because of some deep-seated psychological problems, or perhaps malingering to get attention or to collect insurance money. Although neuropathic pain doesn't always fit the rules of obvious cause and effect, the pain is quite real. It is sometimes so excruciating that it can make someone pull off his clothing to relieve the burning sensation triggered by the touch of cloth on the skin.

Although neuropathic pain affects only 1 percent of the population, it is by far the most potentially debilitating type of pain, physically and psychologically, because of its severity and total unpredictability. It is also the least understood type of pain and the most difficult to treat. However, aside from pain, there are other changes that develop with time when certain neuropathic pain syndromes persist. These include changes in the blood supply to the affected area, with potential deterioration of the nails, skin, muscles, and bones, resulting in further pain and disfigurement. Years of living with constant pain can also lead to chronic personality changes, depression, anger, poverty, divorce, and even suicide. This is a very complex, devastating medical phenomenon.

PAINFUL TWITCH: TRIGEMINAL NEURALGIA

Trigeminal neuralgia, or tic douloureux (painful twitch, in French), is an extremely painful condition involving the fifth cranial, or trigeminal, nerve. This is the most common type of nontraumatic neuralgia in the body. Fortunately, it is still relatively rare, but not rare enough for the fifteen thousand people who develop this disorder in the United States each year. It rarely affects anyone under forty, but it may progress and become more difficult to treat. Many people are in their seventies by the time they seek neurosurgical intervention to control the pain.

The pain produced by this disorder is severe. It is often experienced as a lancinating pain—as if a lance were being stuck repeatedly into the painful area. People often wince during a painful salvo, thus the French name. The neuralgia is almost always associated with a trigger zone— an area of the facial skin which, when stroked lightly or blown by a cold wind, becomes painful. The pain from this condition often progresses with years and eventually may become intractable, with episodes becoming more frequent and increasingly unresponsive to previously effective medication. It exists usually on one side of the face, in the cheek, lips, gums, or chin. Rarely, it can affect the area around the eye and forehead. Even more rarely, it can affect both sides. It affects the right side of the face somewhat more frequently than the left.

Trigeminal neuralgia may be the result of damage to or irritation of the trigeminal nerve or its circuits within the brain or spinal cord. In a few people it is due to conditions such as multiple sclerosis (MS), tumors in or outside the brain, or dilated blood vessels at the base of the brain, which we can find on diagnostic tests like MRI.

In the vast majority, the disease appears for no apparent reason—a form of test-negative pain. Moreover, it can sometimes get better or worse all by itself. I don't mean it goes away, but the need for pain medication may fluctuate over time. And then, in some people, one by one, drugs lose their effectiveness and surgery or other procedures must be considered. As it turns out, they don't necessarily work forever either.

There are twelve cranial nerves that leave the brain at the base of the skull. Certain ones connect with parts of the brain that are a continuation of the spinal cord, bringing sensory information about your environment into the brain for further processing. Three of these nerves—numbers 5, 9, and 10—are implicated in severe neuropathic pain. The fifth transmits sensations from a large area of the front of the head as well as the covering of the brain (the dura) and the blood vessels inside the head. The trigeminal nerve supplies the face, some of the inside of the mouth, and the delicate, transparent covering of the eyes. It also controls the chewing muscles. Most of this trigeminal sensory information goes to specialized areas within the brain. However, incoming painful information goes to the upper few inches of the spinal cord, just below the skull.

The ninth cranial nerve, the glossopharyngeal nerve, carries sensory information from the back of the tongue and mouth, the throat, and part of the ear. It is responsible for some taste sensations and also for the pain you have with an earache or when descending in an airplane. The trigeminal nerve and, far less frequently, the glossopharyngeal nerve, along with their central-nervous-system circuits, may cause tremendous pain or neuralgia (pain arising from a nerve). The tenth, or vagus, nerve also may be involved in glossopharyngeal neuralgia.

Vago-Glossopharyngeal Neuralgia

The ninth nerve, sometimes in association with the tenth nerve, can cause a neuralgia like that of the trigeminal nerve. However, this neuralgia is far less common. Annually, there are approximately 150 new cases of vaso-glossopharyngeal neuralgia in the United States. A few people have both of these cranial neuralgias. As bad as trigeminal neuralgia is, vago-glossopharyngeal neuralgia can be worse. It impairs the ability to eat because it causes shocklike pain at the back of the tongue and in the throat and ear. Like trigeminal neuralgia, it involves only one side of the face, often the left. It may attack the larynx or Adam's apple area, the upper throat, the back of the tongue, and an area deep within the ear. Swallowing, coughing, talking, turning the head, and even touching the ear can cause pain. In the throat, the pain may have an excruciating, electric-shock-like quality. Alternately, the neuralgia may cause a scratchy quality in the throat or the sensation of a bug in the ear.

Treatment with Drugs

The drug Tegretol controls trigeminal neuralgia in at least 75 percent of sufferers and eliminates the need for surgery. Indeed, the diagnosis of trigeminal neuralgia should be questioned in anyone who has not experienced even transient relief on Tegretol. If Tegretol cannot be tolerated,

Dilantin and Depakote are less effective alternatives. If these drugs are ineffective or not tolerated, I add Neurontin to the mix, raising the dose slowly over several weeks to months to avoid sleepiness, the major side effect. Neurontin alone may not give sufficient relief in this condition.

Sometimes Baclofen, a drug normally used to control spasticity, the muscle stiffness seen in cerebral palsy, works well to help control pain from trigeminal neuralgia. I add it to Tegretol or to a multiple-drug regimen of Tegretol and Neurontin, for example. Klonopin, a sister of Valium, may also be effective in combination with other drugs. Mexiletine in some cases has dramatic results. It, too, may be combined in a multiple-drug regimen.

Surgery for the Relief of Trigeminal Neuralgia

The surgical treatment for tic douloureux reflects uncertainty about the cause of this condition. A host of surgical procedures, most of which damage the nerve, its ganglion (a sensory relay station), or nearby root to some degree, have reasonably good effects. Some side effects are potentially severe, including the rare death. Most of these treatments are performed under mild anesthesia by passing needles through the skin of the face along the nerve up close to its origin, just inside a little hole at the base of the skull. In other words, they are "closed," not requiring an incision.

Various "open" surgical techniques exist, and all involve gaining access to the nerve root or its ganglion by entering the skull from the back. These open techniques have included such effective minimalist strategies as just "tweaking" or rubbing the nerve gently with a surgical forceps. More aggressive, and seemingly less effective, strategies involve cutting the sensory nerve roots.

Glycerol Injections and Radiofrequency. The most popular closed procedure today may be the injection of glycerol into the space around the ganglion. Glycerol is injected over the nerve to destroy the nerve tissue. This involves placing a thin needle through the cheek and up through a small hole in the base of the skull, to the area at the base of the brain where the ganglion lies. This is performed in a radiology suite, under intravenous anesthesia, and requires a one-night hospital stay. The effects of the glycerol procedure last two to three years, on average.

The radiofrequency procedure is similar to using glycerol, except that an electrode replaces the needle. The effects of this procedure last significantly longer than the glycerol injection but can result in numbness, including loss of sensation over the covering of the eye. This is a serious problem, resulting in frequent eye inflammations and infections, because of the absence of feeling in the eye. Severe ongoing neuropathic pain—*anesthesia dolorosa,* or painful numbness, a very intractable pain—can occur in the area of numbness.

Glycerol injections present less risk of loss of eye sensation and *anesthesia dolorosa*, although I have seen the latter complication following a glycerol injection.

Microvascular Decompression. In the 1960s, a procedure was devised to separate the nerve from a supposedly irritating artery lying against it. The separation is obtained through the use of a small Teflon patch placed between the nerve and the artery. Usually the offending artery can't be seen except during surgery. Advocates of this approach contend that this sort of artery is a main cause of the problem of trigeminal neuralgia that exists without other cause. The percentage of patients with trigeminal neuralgia who have an abnormal artery pressing on the nerve varies from 11 percent to close to 100 percent, depending on what study you read. This raises a serious question about the above theory. This disease appears to be far more complicated than a little artery pressing on a nerve. Nevertheless, the Teflon advocates have developed quite a following, and the operation, called microvascular decompression, is the major surgical treatment used to treat this condition. The potential hazards of this kind of surgery, although infrequent, are not trivial. Various cranial nerves could be injured and result in stroke, loss of hearing and facial sensation, *anesthesia dolorosa,* permanent loss of balance, and even death.

There are pros and cons to the above procedures. If you are contemplating a procedure to relieve your pain, find someone with experience and a good track record in treating trigeminal neuralgia, using a procedure with which they are comfortable and familiar. Better yet, find more than one physician and compare notes.

Most of the above "long-acting" procedures have an initial 85 to 98 percent success rate. Over ten years, 20 to 50 percent of those treated may suffer again. Any significant recurrence rate undermines the theory behind microvascular decompression. Moreover, second and third procedures—no matter which kind—may be less helpful. No matter what is done, some people will relapse, perhaps more than once.

Radiation Therapy. In the past decade, pencil-point-beam radiation therapy has been applied to the trigeminal nerve just as it leaves the brain, in the hopes of destroying enough nerve to control the pain.

This technique, initially introduced in the early 1950s, is considered an alternative to surgery or other procedures and has been highly successful and well tolerated with few side effects. This procedure should be evaluated carefully over time. It may best be reserved for older patients. One long-term side effect of radiation is the far-delayed occurrence of radiation-induced tumors, which are often malignant.

A Tangled Mass of Nerves: Neuromas

Peripheral nerves resemble an insulated fiber-optic cable in which each of the nerve fibers is separated by a sheath of insulating material. Nerves in the skin and around the muscles are cut during every operation and in everyday trauma, such as when you cut yourself with a kitchen knife. In most cases, the severed nerve regenerates and may grow back into the same approximate area. No soreness or numbness occurs once the nerve heals or nearby nerves take over some of the function of the damaged nerve.

In some cases, however, nerves may not regrow properly but instead form a tangled mass of sprouting nerve fibers, only partially covered with insulating material. This mass is called a neuroma and may act like a short circuit and become a source of severe pain. Pain from these nerve sprouts may exist spontaneously when skin over them is tapped or nearby muscles are contracted.

It is not clear why some people develop neuromas from a given trauma and others do not. Most of us go through life with all sorts of cuts, some of which even become infected, and undergo major surgical procedures, usually without neuroma formation. Nerves in certain locations may be more predisposed to damage and possible neuroma formation than others. Following thoracic surgery, in which incisions are made between the ribs to expose the lungs or heart, neuromas of the little nerves under the ribs seem to occur with greater likelihood than in other areas. This may be due to the anatomy of the chest. In the chest, the nerves under the ribs may be compressed between two hard surfaces—the surgical instrument that pries open the ribs and the ribs themselves. In the abdomen, however, the surgical retractor that holds open the nerves presses against the relatively soft muscles of the abdominal wall. Nerves under the retractor are cushioned by the surrounding muscles, reducing the risk of damage during surgical retraction. Preventing the formation of neuromas is vitally important, as neurons can be difficult to diagnose and treat.

The Man with the Painful Scar That Interfered with Sex

Richard Choi had a painful scar following a routine right-sided hernia operation. He was an advertising executive and his sedentary position did not provoke pain during most of the day. However, it interfered with his ability to perform strenuous exercise, especially on the weekends, as well as play with his young son. Occasionally, it caused pain during or after sexual intercourse. Repeated evaluations by urologists and general surgeons failed to find anything other than a small spot of pain within the scar from his hernia surgery. A general surgeon sent him to me for a pain-relieving procedure.

The skin over and around the scar, just above the crease between the abdomen and thigh and just to the right of the pubic hair, felt perfectly normal. Richard felt excruciating pain if the painful spot—smaller than the tip of my finger—was probed directly with the tip of a Q-tip. However, the pain was not on the surface of the skin but deeper down, suggesting it arose from the covering of the muscles of the abdomen. Tapping the area firmly produced a sharp, localized pain. I believed Richard had an area of pain deep within the otherwise painless scar, possibly a neuroma of a nerve in his lower abdomen. Or perhaps a nerve was wrapped under a suture and thus constantly irritated. I explained that a neuroma really must be diagnosed by cutting out the painful area and examining it with a microscope. Although the operation could totally relieve the pain, surgery of this type may create other pain and even more neuromas. He was not interested in chasing the diagnosis with a knife and agreed with my strategy to try to control his pain with medication first and consider surgery only if the medication was not effective. Pamelor (nortriptyline), a tricyclic antidepressant, was quite helpful. However, it impaired his sexual function. We then tried an anticonvulsant, Neurontin (gabapentin), that worked but made him sleepy. After several months of trial and error with a few other anticonvulsants, he still obtained pain relief only at the expense of some minor but annoying side effects, which prompted him to ask me to try to relieve his pain through a procedure.

I blocked the site of the pain by using a nerve stimulator to help find the area with the greatest pain, then delivering a very small amount of anesthetic to that site. This procedure demonstrated that his pain came from the surface of the muscles making up the abdominal wall. It also temporarily relieved his pain and supported, but did not prove, the concept that he had a neuroma.

Freezing the painful area with cryoanalgesia worked for a month, but he was not interested in repeating this procedure on his groin. I explained to him that I could try to block the nerve root in his spine that supplied the painful part of his abdomen. He agreed, the block was carried out with a local anesthetic, and the results were excellent. In order to create a more long-lasting block, I would use radiofrequency to heat and selectively lesion the ganglion of the spinal root involved in bringing pain impulses from his abdomen to the spinal cord. I explained to him that I had applied this technique to many patients with his type of painful scar, often successfully and occasionally unsuccessfully, but without any long-term side effects. However, in theory, this treatment could also worsen his pain. He still was interested in proceeding with the treatment.

Using meticulous technique and the help of a CAT scanner to guide the placement of my electrode over the ganglion, which lay a short distance from the spinal cord, I performed a radiofrequency lesion of the ganglion. It worked and his pain has not returned in two and a half years. I will never know if he had a true neuroma or not, but I am pleased that I was able to provide him with long-term relief of his pain.

DIABETIC NEUROPATHY

Neuropathies are disorders in which peripheral nerve fibers are damaged by local trauma; exposure to toxins, such as chemotherapy; or a systemic disease like diabetes. Neuropathies may involve both sides of the body equally, beginning in the lower legs and eventually creeping up the legs and affecting the arms. In other cases, individual cranial or peripheral nerves may be affected. Diabetic neuropathy is the most common form of disabling, painful neuropathy in the world. (Leprosy may be the cause of the most common neuropathy, but it is not painful.) It is also the most common example of a metabolic disorder causing neuropathic pain. About 60 percent of people who have had diagnosed diabetes for more than twenty-five years have some form of neuropathy, with or without symptoms, and about 10 percent experience pain.

Numbness and tingling in the feet are often the first sign of diabetic neuropathy. Symptoms are slight at first, and since most nerve damage occurs over a period of years, mild cases may go unnoticed for a long time. Later, a deep, burning pain, worse at night, may affect the feet and legs on both sides. Sufferers may also experience supersensitivity of the skin overlying the affected feet and lower legs. This condition usually progresses slowly. There may be damage to one nerve, usually in the arm or leg, or one of the cranial nerves, causing pain and weakness. This kind of diabetic damage may come on slowly or suddenly, like a stroke. In fact, in certain cases it may represent a stroke of the affected nerve. A common form of this neuropathy affects the nerve in the front of the thigh that controls the muscles that straighten the knee. Once it is damaged, there is sharp, severe pain in the front of the thigh, along with some knee weakness. This type of diabetic nerve damage improves with time.

Another condition, called diabetic amyotrophy, results in wasting of the muscles of the upper legs, with resultant pain in the thighs and lumbar area, usually worse at night. Numbness is not a prominent feature of this kind of diabetic neuropathy. Finally, diabetes can attack the autonomic nerves. This doesn't result in pain but can cause problems with internal organs and cause digestive, heart, or sexual problems.

Diabetics also develop advanced artherosclerosis and poor circulation in their legs. If they develop cuts or sores in their feet, they may not heal and may later become infected. They may also become gangrenous due to poor blood supply.

Given this setup for potential disaster, pressure put on certain areas of the foot from tight shoes may result in foot ulcers. Loss of sensation in the feet can mean that injuries go unnoticed and untreated, and become infected. If ulcers or foot injuries are not treated in time, the infection may progress, even involving the bone. Some infections may lead to amputation; but if caught in time and proper hygiene is practiced, these problems can be controlled.

Treating the Pain of Diabetic Neuropathy

Treatment of diabetic neuropathy is focused first on relieving the pain, second on preventing further damage. Treating the pain involves the usual drugs for neuropathic pain. These drugs are associated with some troublesome side effects, and those with diabetic neuropathy are often elderly and may also have bad hearts and kidneys, which makes the use of many drugs more difficult. Any pain regimen, therefore, must be applied through a stepwise approach, matching an individual's pain requirements and general health to the drug regimen.

For any painful neuropathy, tricyclic antidepressants have definitely demonstrated benefit. They should be considered first, before other drugs. I would consider Pamelor or Norpramin, unless you have heart-rhythm disturbances, glaucoma, or an enlarged prostate, any of which could result in complications with these drugs. Other tricyclics may be tried as well. Tricyclics are inexpensive, safe, and easy to take and therefore I often prescribe them first.

If needed, I add anticonvulsants to tricyclics, or use them instead of the tricyclics in certain patients. Anticonvulsants such as Neurontin, Tegretol, and Dilantin may be used with success. Neurontin, which is quite safe and requires no blood tests, is more expensive than many other drugs in its class, but is generally well tolerated and has been shown to benefit painful diabetic neuropathy. Dilantin may be taken once daily. Tegretol and Neurontin need to be taken several times daily. Both Dilantin and Tegretol require blood testing on a regular basis.

Mexitil, a drug that controls the heart rhythm, can be used possibly in conjunction with the above drugs. It should be reserved for patients with otherwise poorly controlled pain. It cannot be used if you have certain kinds of heart disease, and it requires monitoring of the blood and EKG. Sometimes a phenothiazine (a potent psychiatric drug, one of the most commonly prescribed types of drugs in the United States), may be considered. Other drugs have been used with varying success, including non-narcotic analgesics, such as Ultram. Capsaicin topical cream (Zostrix) can also be rubbed on for pain relief.

At the same time, blood-sugar levels must be brought under control by diet, oral drugs, or insulin, and carefully monitored. Some studies show that tight control of blood sugar may renew lost sensation, and possibly help prevent or delay further problems.

THE NEUROPATHIC PAIN SYNDROMES OF AIDS/HIV

Distal Symmetrical Polyneuropathies (DSPN) are perhaps the most common type of neuropathic pain syndrome occurring among HIV patients. After abdominal pain, peripheral neuropathy is the second most common source of all pain in HIV disease, occurring in about 25 percent of patients. A study in the *New England Journal of Medicine* in 1994 categorizes the intensity of pain in HIV disease as comparable to cancer pain. Obviously, as the disease advances, the pain increases.

Distal means farthest away from the center of the body, as in hands and feet. DSPN can result from either the infection itself, from alcohol use, or as a result of a vitamin B deficiency (B_2, B_6, and B_{12}). It is also a side effect of many HIV/AIDS drugs, such as zalcitabine (Hivid), stavudine (Zerit), and didanosine (Didex). Symptoms of DSPN include foot pain and weakness as well as decreased sensation in the feet. As the name implies, DSPN occurs symmetrically, in both feet, and affects many ("poly") sensory nerves.

The cause of painful neuropathy in HIV infection is unknown. One theory proposes a viral cause, and a 1997 study demonstrated direct viral invasion of peripheral nerves. Despite this theory, antiviral therapy can worsen painful neuropathy and possibly even cause it, further muddying the waters.

The new antiviral drugs used to combat AIDS may cause some neuropathy but are exceedingly effective at keeping the disease in check. Although AIDS-related neuropathic pain is still a significant clinical problem, excruciating pain now seems less common. However, there are a wide variety of different types of neuropathic pain that can occur in people with HIV disease or full-blown AIDS.

Treatment with Drugs

As with cancer, pain relief should be a major focus of treatment, but advanced AIDS presents special challenges. For example, gastrointestinal disorders such as diarrhea, malabsorption, and difficulty swallowing (dysphagia) present problems with oral medication, so alternate delivery methods (described in chapter 3) are sometimes needed. The treatment of this neuropathy is similar to that of diabetes.

If anticonvulsants are needed, I prefer Neurontin for this patient population. Unlike the other anticonvulsants, it is unlikely to damage the blood, liver, or kidneys, which may already be impaired in someone with AIDS. The antidepressants and antiarrythmics (sodium channel blockers) should be used with caution in people who have preexisting heart disease or mental changes due to the effect of AIDS on the brain. These drugs may worsen or cause certain cardiac problems as well as agitation or confusion. Tramadol and narcotics may also exacerbate or cause confusion, especially in these patients.

AIDS patients may already be taking other medication which can harm their liver, or they may have coexisting hepatitis with liver damage. Acetaminophen, a common ingredient in many pain preparations, can harm the liver. Therefore, acetaminophen (Tylenol), or pain relievers containing this drug—Tylenol with codeine, Vicodin, or Percoset, for example—should be given with caution to patients with liver damage. This includes those with or without AIDS. Other narcotic medications, without acetaminophen, can be used, if needed, with good pain relieving effects.

Pain in AIDS patients *can* and *should* be controlled. The effects of advanced AIDS on the body just makes pain management in these patients more challenging. It is the duty of physicians and other care providers to accept that challenge with expertise, creativity, and compassion.

COMPLEX REGIONAL PAIN SYNDROME (CRPS): THE BLACK HOLE OF NEUROPATHIC PAIN

What the medical profession now calls complex regional pain syndrome (CRPS)—a mouthful by any standard—was only recently changed from the previous name, reflex sympathetic dystrophy (RSD). Before that, this strange disorder was called by twelve other names, including minor causalgia and shoulder–hand syndrome. This musical-chairs game of names reflects the confusion surrounding the cause and treatment of this serious but enigmatic disorder. These names also reflect the unusual and sometimes dramatic tissue changes seen in the affected extremity.

The phenomenon was first described by a group of surgeons during the Civil War. (One of these doctors, S. Weir Mitchell, also described phantom-limb pain.) The doctors noticed that some soldiers with severe pain from hand or foot injuries would fill their boots with water or wrap their affected limbs in wet rags to "extinguish the fire." Dr. Mitchell named the condition causalgia, from the Greek *kausos* (heat) and *algos* (pain) in 1867. This checkered history surrounding CRPS leaves no doubt that it is a kind of black hole of neuropathic pain.

The International Association for the Study of Pain (IASP) recently classified two different types of CRPS. Type 1, the syndrome formerly called RSD, does not involve obvious injury to the peripheral nervous system. Its deep, diffuse pain is brought on by infection, inflammation, surgery, heart attack, stroke, degenerative joint disease, burns, or prolonged nerve compression following the use of a plaster cast, to name but a few of its causes. Diagnosis is made five to six weeks after the onset of pain, because after this time injury to other tissues should have resolved. In contrast, Type II (formerly called causalgia) results from obvious peripheral nerve injury. In CRPS Type II, the areas of the body most often affected are the hand and foot, but pain can spread to involve the entire limb as well as unrelated structures. In about 85 percent of cases of CRPS Type II the pain persists for more than six months; in about 25 percent of cases it continues for one year or more.

Old studies suggest that CRPS rarely occurs in people under sixteen, appears to be more common in Caucasians, and is three times more common in women than men. In up to 15 percent of people, this disorder may follow trauma, with psychological factors playing an influential role in bringing it on.

The case of Maryann Dart exemplifies the terrible nature of this disorder. Ten years ago, a steel door crushed the fingers of Ms. Dart's right hand. Four years and three surgeries later, she was finally diagnosed with reflex sympathetic dystrophy (as CRPS was then known) that continued to spread. Following several briefly successful blocks of the sympathetic nerves to her affected right hand, she had a sympathectomy, a procedure that interrupts the presumed painful hyperactivity of the sympathetic nervous system with chemicals, heat, or surgery. The procedure produced no long-term benefit, and her pain continued. She has become totally disabled and is now confined to a wheelchair. The pain has spread to her pelvis and groin, left hand, and left leg. It has affected the muscles of her eyes, causing a visual problem, and also affects her esophagus and bladder. The intensity of her pain is reduced while she is in warm water. She frequently goes to a warm swimming pool for some relief.

As in the case of Ms. Dart, people with CRPS often suffer through months, even years, of failed treatments before a true diagnosis is made and more appropriate therapy is begun. This frustrating course of trial and error reflects the many faces of the disease, particularly in its early stages. It can look like many other kinds of nerve pain from many different types of injuries and conditions, not to mention psychiatric disease. In up to 10 percent of cases there appears to be no obvious cause.

Symptoms

While the initial causes of the two types of CRPS may differ, the conditions have similar features, such as the horrible continuous pain in the affected areas, usually the extremities. The pain may feel like intense burning, occasionally in combination with an acute stabbing sensation. Some people describe *knifelike, piercing*, and *throbbing pain*, as well as *deep aching*. These flare-ups are out of proportion to the most innocuous stimuli, such as a breeze, a noise, moving an arm, or feeling anxious. A quick touch can set off a half hour of increased burning pain. The central nervous system is clearly hyperexcited or hypersensitized. Moreover, the distribution of the pain often doesn't follow the distribution of peripheral nerves, suggesting that the cause and mechanism for continuation and eventual spread of the pain involves more than the peripheral nervous system. The central nervous system may be important in the spread of this disorder.

Painful areas become swollen, red, warm, and dry. Later in the disease, the skin becomes sweaty, shiny, blue, and cold, and the nails get dry and cracked. The joints become stiff and fixed in contracted positions. Hands assume clawlike positions, muscles shrink, and the bones begin to lose calcium and become osteoporotic. Finally, the disease spreads up the limbs toward the central body. This process may involve limbs on the other side or even other parts of the body. Severe deformity of the affected extremities results in total physical and mental disability. The changes in the soft tissues and bones are thought to be caused first by augmented blood supply and later by diminished blood supply, presumably due to abnormal sympathetic nervous system activity.

Pain Management with Sympathetic Nerve Blockades

The management of CRPS usually involves a stepwise approach that depends largely on the severity and progression of the condition. All therapy is combined with active rehabilitation. Medication for neuropathic pain (anticonvulsants), tricyclic antidepressants, certain antiarrythmics, narcotics, and even oral corticosteroids have been effective in relieving pain in CRPS. However, CRPS is considered by some to be a special type of neuropathic pain, caused or complicated by overactivity of the sympathetic nervous system.

The sympathetic nerves travel with other nerves out of the spine, but their major role is not sensation or movement but controlling bodily functions, like blood flow and sweating, for example. Sympathetic nerves, when they fire, cause the muscles in blood vessel walls to tighten, which constricts the vessels, so less blood can flow through them. A limb affected by sympathetic overdrive could become cold and blue. If these nerves are at rest—not firing—the vessels they control open up, allowing more blood to flow into the limb, making it warm and pink. Blocking the sympathetic nerves with a local anesthetic will result in dilation of blood vessels, increasing blood flow and warming of the area supplied by the blocked nerves. In the block, the anesthetic is injected directly onto sympathetic ganglia, relay centers of the sympathetic nervous system. These are located next to the front of the spine in the neck, upper thorax, and lumbar area.

For those who believe CRPS is due to excessive sympathetic activity, reducing this overactivity should relieve pain and reverse disability. A sympathetic block results in a temporary, and a sympathectomy in a long-term, interruption of sympathetic nerve impulses supplying an area, such as an arm.

Sympathetic nerve blocks often provide pain relief for about three to four hours. The blocks may be repeated at regular intervals, with the goal of progressively dampening a vicious cycle of sympathetic nervous activity and pain. Unfortunately, the response to these blocks may vary even in the same person and there is also the risk of perforation of major blood vessels or other structures, such as the lung, depending on where they are performed.

If sympathetic blocks provide short- but not long-term relief, a sympathectomy may be considered.

Chemical sympathectomy is the injection of chemicals toxic to nerves, such as phenol or alcohol, onto the appropriate sympathetic nerves. *Radiofrequency* may be used to destroy the sympathetic nerves. Both chemical and radiofrequency techniques may last several months and can be repeated. *Surgical procedures* involve the removal of a piece of the sympathetic nervous system, producing a much longer lasting result.

Intravenous regional sympathetic blockade is a less invasive approach in which the affected limb is isolated with a tourniquet and a drug such as guanethidine is injected into the veins. Guanethidine inhibits or blocks sympathetic activity. The drug accumulates in a high local concentration during the twenty to thirty minutes the limb is wrapped in the tourniquet, so its antisympathetic effect is localized. More recently this treatment has been called into question and found in some studies to be no more effective than a placebo (saline injection), but it may be more effective when given early in the condition. An alternative approach to therapy, which appears to have had positive results, is the delivery of guanethidine through the skin of the affected area. This is done using a gentle electrical stimulation.

Unfortunately, these procedures all too often do not provide long-term pain relief (see below).

Oral Drug Therapy

Following the logic underlying the previous procedures, to the extent that the sympathetic nervous system is involved in the pain and secondary effects of CRPS, oral medication may be used to block sympathetic-nervous-system activity. These drugs include some that are ordinarily used to lower blood pressure in people with hypertension. Some drugs diminish the activity of the sympathetic nervous system by blocking the ability of norepinephrine, a neurotransmitter of this system, to bind to certain receptors. Drugs such as Inderal (propranolol), in dosages up to 320 mg daily, are prescribed to CRPS patients. Inderal can block the early-warning effects of low blood sugar and should not be given to diabetics being treated with oral medication or insulin. It also can worsen asthma. Other potential side effects of propranolol include low blood pressure, depression, feeling weak or faint due to low blood pressure, and impotence or inability to ejaculate. Drugs that block other receptors in the sympathetic nervous system include Minipress (prazosin) and Dibenzyline (phenoxybenzamine).

Another drug works by stimulating, not blocking, yet another type of sympathetic-nervous-system receptors and paradoxically reduces, rather than stimulates, sympathetic activity. Catapress (clonidine), which is given as a skin patch, works in this fashion. All these drugs can make you feel weak or faint, because they lower your blood pressure whether or not they provide pain relief.

Another type of drug that works on the heart and blood vessels, Procardia (nifedipine), is also sometimes used in CRPS Type I patients. Procardia is a type of drug called a peripheral calcium channel blocker, which dilates the blood vessels and is thus effective in treating the aspects of CRPS attributed to decreased blood supply to an affected area.

Other Treatments for CRPS

For some severe cases, indwelling pumps or spinal-cord stimulation, mentioned later in this chapter, may help significantly. These measures provide pain relief so that physical therapy can be used to restore function to the affected limb. Even with treatment, symptoms remain present in up to 60 percent of people suffering from CRPS.

The Placebo Effect

Most if not all of the success of blocking or destroying sympathetic nerves in CRPS may be attributable to the placebo effect. Up to 60 percent of people with this disease respond for a short period to this scientifically questionable intervention. The placebo effect is the link between the mind and the body. Suggestion may cause the effect, but the body produces the pain relief underlying the effect. The naturally occurring opioid system appears to be involved in the placebo response. The placebo effect is partially blocked by drugs that interfere with the effect of narcotics—including the body's natural opioids. Also, anxiety, which often accompanies pain, makes pain worse, possibly by creating further spasm in muscles already tight from ongoing pain, among other things. Belief in a new treatment may reduce anxiety, relax tight muscles, and partially relieve pain. It is unethical and scientifically inappropriate to use placebos to determine whether or not your pain is real. A positive response to a water injection is a real effect and cannot differentiate real pain from fake. In fact, people with the worst pain are the most likely to respond to a placebo. Anyone can experience a placebo effect under the right circumstances. If one hundred people in pain are given a "very special pain reliever" (really water), at least thirty of them will note a real, temporary reduction in pain. The more they are in pain, the more they want a treatment to work, and the more they believe in the potential of the treatment to work, the more likely it is that a placebo effect will occur.

CRPS should be recognized and treated, like other neuropathic painful disorders, by competent pain specialists as early as possible so as to minimize the risk of sensitization of the central nervous system. The role for invasive and even pharmacological manipulations of the sympathetic nervous system, as opposed to other means of pain control in CRPS, must be further clarified.

Pain Following Shingles: Postherpetic Neuralgia

Postherpetic neuralgia is a complication of herpes zoster (shingles) occurring in up to 15 percent of people who develop shingles. This pain lasts a month or more after the attack of shingles is over. It is probably one of the most common forms of neuropathic pain and occurs in at least one in ten adults aged forty or older and about half of the people over sixty who develop shingles. Most people recover from postherpetic neuralgia, although the recovery rate diminishes with age. At one year, pain from postherpetic neuralgia resolves in about 80 percent of those over age fifty-five, but only in 50 percent of people over seventy.

The pain of postherpetic neuralgia is variably described as spasms of shooting, stabbing pain or burning, or as a severe deep aching sensation in the affected area (most commonly on the thorax). There also might be a loss of feeling in the affected area or such extreme skin sensitivity that brushing a piece of clothing against the skin can cause sharp pain. Pain can also occur spontaneously. The source of pain is damage to peripheral nerves and the spinal cord. In either case, the pain-transmitting neurons within the spinal cord may be overactive.

Herpes zoster is an infection caused by the same virus that causes chicken pox. It is one of the most common infectious diseases affecting the nervous system, most often occurring in people over the age of fifty. (Herpes simplex, causing fever blisters and genital herpes, may be more common.) The chance of developing zoster increases with age, and is associated with a significant falloff in immunity, especially marked after age sixty. From ages fifty to seventy, up to one person in one hundred may develop zoster. By age eighty, up to one in three people may experience the disease. Patients with impaired immunity due to medications, HIV infection, or cancer, especially leukemia or lymphoma, are also particularly likely to develop herpes zoster. A popular explanation given for why and how herpes zoster develops is that it results from a reactivation of the chicken-pox or varicella-zoster virus lying dormant in those who have had chicken pox earlier in life. Herpes zoster occurs in 15 percent of people who have had chicken pox. Some of the chicken-pox virus lodges itself in the nervous system, lying dormant. Years later, age, illness, or stress can reactivate the remaining virus.

Painful, supersensitive areas of skin may temporarily be made pain-free in some cases by injecting the area with local anesthetic. The local anesthetic simply blocks the transmission of peripheral pain messages to the spinal cord. These blocks may temporarily relieve pain from damaged peripheral nerves. However, some people with postherpetic neuralgia have damaged spinal cords and respond abnormally to any sensation—and they may even have spontaneous pain.

Autopsies of people who have had postherpetic neuralgia showed abnormal changes in the dorsal-root entry zone (see figure 1, page 6), the area where the peripheral nerves deliver their pain impulses to the spinal cord. Blocks of peripheral nerves will have no effect if pain results from spinal-cord damage.

The terrible physical pain of postherpetic neuralgia is only part of the problem. The psychological pain resulting from the difficulty of treating this condition affects not only the sufferer but virtually everyone touched by him or her. Spouses, children and physicians alike become frustrated by the difficulty of successfully treating this condition.

Treatment of Postherpetic Neuralgia

There is still no consensus among clinicians about how to manage acute herpes zoster, but it is generally believed that it is important to treat the infection as early as possible. The *New England Journal of*

Medicine reported in 1996 that treatment within seventy-two hours of developing the rash can reduce the severity of the infection. Such treatment also may help reduce the length and severity of postherpetic neuralgia that may later develop, or may even prevent it, but this is still unclear. However, the recommended treatments for postherpetic neuralgia (at one month or more after the initial herpes zoster) are more numerous and less clear-cut than those for herpes zoster itself. Their effectiveness varies widely from one person to another.

Drug approaches include the use of a tricyclic antidepressant and/or anticonvulsants. The anticonvulsant gabapentin (Neurontin) may be the best drug for the initial treatment of many neuropathic pain disorders in the elderly. It is safe, and if the dose is raised slowly enough, the major side effect—sedation—usually doesn't occur. When prescribed for postherpetic neuralgia, tricyclic antidepressants are given in smaller dosages than they are for depression. These drugs may work best for deep aching pain. Although they don't eliminate the pain, they make it easier to deal with it. Long- and short-acting narcotics may be used in conjunction with the above drugs.

Drugs such as major tranquilizers (perphenazine, or Trilafon), the Valium-like drug clonazepam (Klonopin), the blood-pressure medication clonidine (Minipress), and mexiletine (Mexitil) may be considered as well. Unfortunately, the very elderly who are most likely to suffer from intractable postherpetic neuralgia are also those least likely to tolerate the complicated drug regimens needed to control the pain of the neuralgia.

Topical Treatment. Fortunately, topical analgesic and anesthetic creams such as lidocaine-prilocaine cream or 5 percent lidocaine gel often work well, at least for a while. These may be helpful, particularly for people with supersensitive skin. Capsaicin cream (Zostrix) may also help, but is often not tolerated due to the burning sensation produced by the chili-pepper-derived cream.

Other therapies, such as transcutaneous electrical nerve stimulation (TENS), hypnosis, biofeedback, and psychosocial or behavioral techniques can complement the traditional medical treatments. (These are outlined in chapter 2.) In some cases, spinal-cord stimulation, implantable pumps for delivery of intraspinal analgesics, and various neurosurgical interventions may be considered to provide pain relief.

The best way to prevent postherpetic neuralgia may be to prevent the herpes zoster infection itself. A new vaccine is available against varicella, but we still do not know whether it will prevent the later development of herpes zoster. Vaccination of those over sixty with an appropriate vaccine designed to boost their immunity to the varicella zoster virus is currently being investigated.

THE SPIDER'S PAINFUL WEB: ARACHNOIDITIS

Arachnoiditis is a scarring of the arachnoid or spiderweblike inner covering of the spinal cord. It may result from some form of chemical that comes into contact with the arachnoid during an intraspinal injection and starts an inflammation of this covering. This causes scarring to varying degrees. This scarring mats the roots to each other, making them vulnerable to being tugged on with every body movement. The scarring presumably also interferes with blood flow in tiny blood vessels that supply the roots, causing some nerve fibers to function poorly if at all. The damaged fibers may cause pain, numbness, or weakness of the legs as well as sexual, urinary, and rectal dysfunction.

The prime suspect of this chemical insult is a radiological dye—Pantopaque—that was used for myelograms in the past. This was injected into the spinal fluid and came into contact with the arachnoid. In most cases there were no ill effects or it caused some arachnoiditis with few symptoms. However, for some unfortunate people, it resulted in progressive pain and neurological dysfunction from the slow, inexorable scarring of the arachnoid as it came into contact with the dye. Another past cause was the intentional injection of steroids into the spinal fluid for treatment of nerve-root pain from disk herniation, or to control the symptoms during flare-ups of multiple sclerosis.

Focal arachnoiditis exists around all areas in which the central nervous system was invaded surgically, but this form of the condition causes no ill effects. It is the diffuse progressive form that causes the problem, because it involves the cauda equina, the bundle of nerves in the lower spine. Pain from this kind of arachnoiditis can never be completely eradicated, no matter what is done. In the past, physicians have been known to try to cut away the scar tissue, but this usually makes the condition worse.

Pain can be controlled using drugs commonly used for neuropathic pain as well as narcotics given by mouth or in skin patches. The spinal-cord stimulators described on page 156 are also helpful. Alternatively, pain medication delivered into the spinal fluid by an implanted pump may be considered.

PAIN FROM DAMAGED NERVE ROOTS

When the fibers of the spinal nerve roots are severed, the pain-transmitting nerve cells in the cord to which the roots formerly brought sensory impulses become hyperactive, firing willy-nilly and producing pain when there is no reason to experience pain. This kind of pain may subside with time, or may require chronic treatment. It is very common in the building trades, where workers fall from scaffolding and other high places, and also among veterans injured by shrapnel. I once had the challenge of treating the survivor of a near-fatal fall. Unfortunately, when I met thirty-nine-year-old Mr. Stoneblood six months after his accident, he was in so much pain that he wished he had not survived.

The Man Who Fell off the Roof

Mr. Stoneblood, a roofer, had been installing a slate roof on a three-story house when he slipped from the top of the roof, sliding down the side. He went flying toward the edge and probable death. But as he slipped into space, he managed to grasp onto a piece of scaffolding a story below and break his fall with his right arm. He could not hold on and fell, but hit a pile of tarps on the ground below.

Mr. Stoneblood was severely bruised, smashed an ankle, and had a mild concussion. At the hospital, it was noted that his right arm was quite weak and that he was numb over part of his shoulder, arm, and hand. His spine was not broken and his brain was unharmed. His broken ankle was repaired surgically and he was evaluated by a neurologist who felt that he had damaged the nerves that supply the arm, called the brachial plexus.

The hospital had no MRI, so the doctor ordered a CAT scan and myelogram of Mr. Stoneblood's neck. The myelogram explained the weakness and numbness. Mr. Stoneblood had suffered a brachial plexus avulsion—that is, some of the nerve roots that leave the spinal cord in the neck and supply the shoulder, arm, and hand had been ripped out of the spinal cord when he tried to break his fall. He would never completely regain the lost function or feeling of his right arm again. Over the next few weeks, he began to develop horrible chronic burning pain and pins-and-needles sensations in the areas of numbness. He also suffered from spontaneous episodes of excruciating, shooting pain in the arm, radiating up to the shoulder.

Mr. Stoneblood was treated with tricyclic antidepressants and anticonvulsants that provided little relief. When he came to me, I explained that this kind of pain was due to hyperactive nerve cells in his spinal cord that were firing at random and producing pain for no apparent reason. Likewise, the fibers exiting the cord and governing movement were also severed, making him weak. I explained that this kind of pain may subside with time, or may require chronic treatment, but he would remain weak and numb to some extent.

In the meantime, I tried him on various drug cocktails that reduced his pain about 40 percent. He had previously done poorly in rehabilitation because of his pain. With the modest pain reduction from the medication, he was able to relearn how to use his weakened arm to maximal benefit, but he still was quite incapacitated by pain. He was also quite emphatic that he could live with his weakness and numbness but could not conceive of going through the remainder of his life in this kind of pain. He agreed to try other forms of treatment.

A trial of spinal-cord stimulation failed, as did intraspinal pain medication. What eventually worked was a neurosurgical procedure called a DREZ lesion. This operation destroys the dorsal-root entry zone (DREZ), where the axons of the peripheral nerves enter the spinal cord and connect with the pain pathway. This operation achieved a remarkable, sustained control of Mr. Stoneblood's pain. Sometimes nature is kind to us. Cutting out a bad chip in the most complex computer known to man can be tremendously helpful. Moreover, certain chips may be removed without causing the whole system to crash.

STROKE OR SPINAL-CORD-INJURY PAIN

When parts of the brain or spinal cord are damaged by a stroke, neuropathic pain can result. Central-nervous-system pain occurs in 2 to 8 percent of all stroke cases, in at least 20 percent of strokes involving the side and back of the thalamus, and in 25 to 40 percent of spinal-cord injuries. Pain is caused either by irritation of the pain-impulse-carrying fibers (organized in a bundle called a tract) or damage to fibers that inhibit pain-impulse traffic within this tract. The same medications used for other neuropathic pain conditions can be used to treat pain from stroke or spinal-cord injury.

The Pain from Out of the Blue

Maggie Jones is a patient with an unfortunately placed hole—a result of a small stroke—in her brain that causes terrible burning pain over her lower leg and, to a lesser extent, her forearm opposite to the side of the hole. Ms. Jones experienced the most common cause of central-nervous-system damage—stroke. She had a long history of high blood pressure, for which she took medicine, but otherwise was healthy.

One day, out of the blue, she developed burning pain over one side of her body, particularly affecting the right forearm and hand but especially her lower leg. It was as if the heat of fire was switched on suddenly. The burning was associated with no other complaints initially. She went to her family doctor the next day and he found nothing wrong. A week later, she developed low-back pain. The family doctor referred her to a neurologist who evaluated her for various disorders that could cause this kind of pain, including multiple sclerosis, as well as diseases of her spinal cord and nerve roots, all without any result. He concluded that she must have had a small stroke due to her hypertension, and closer examination of her MRI showed a small hole over the back and side of the thalamus. This hole represented the effect of a tiny stroke.

PHANTOM-LIMB PAIN

Nearly everyone who has an amputation has a phantom-limb sensation. They feel as if their missing limb is still there. This sensation is more common than most people realize, and so is very real pain from the phantom limb. Such pain is described as shooting, sharp, lancinating, burning, crushing, or cramping. The pain may be continuous or intermittent. It may be provoked or aggravated by movement of the stump or by heat. This pain usually subsides as time passes. Stump pain at the site of the amputation is different from phantom-limb pain. Stump pain persists long after the stump is healed and is very difficult to treat.

Phantom-limb pain usually starts soon after amputation but could appear weeks, months, or even years later. The pain can be occasional and mild, or continuous and severe. A typical complaint in phantom-hand pain is the feeling that the hand is clenched, fingers bent over the thumb and digging into the palm so that the whole hand is tired and achy. In phantom-leg pain, the discomfort may feel like a cramp in the calf. Many other amputees report feeling as if their toes are being seared by a red-hot poker. People can have a phantom-limb pain even when the limb is not completely severed, when it is paralyzed, or when the spinal cord is anesthetized.

The earliest explanation for phantom-limb pain was that the nerves in the stump develop neuromas, which continue to generate pain impulses that flow up through the spinal cord to the brain. Using this theory as a rationale for treatment, researchers and clinicians have tried to stop the transmission of pain impulses at each of these levels. They have cut the nerves around the stump, usually just above the neuroma or at the roots, or just before the nerves enter the spinal cord. They also have severed pathways within the spinal cord as well as in areas of the thalamus within the brain. Such invasive approaches do not abolish the phantom limb, but they can provide some relief of pain for months, even years, although the pain usually returns. Other theories implicate the spinal cord as being responsible for phantom-limb pain and claim that neuromas have nothing to do with it. Still other theories propose the circuitry of the brain as the basis for phantom-limb pain.

One likely explanation holds that the brain contains an imprint of the entire body, which may be present from birth and is modified by life's experiences. Under this theory, when a limb is amputated, the neural circuitry containing the central imprint of the intact body remains. The phantom limb is still perceived as being part of the body. The usual incoming sensory signals from the amputated limb concerning its position in space, the tightness of its muscles, and pain obviously disappear after the amputation.

However, it appears that after loss of a limb, new circuits grow or previously unused circuits become active within the brain—underscoring the ability of the central nervous system to grow or change, even in fully formed adults. These new connections may connect the brain areas that previously processed information from the lost limb to nearby brain areas receiving sensory information from another still-intact part of the body. So impulses from the hand or face, stimulated by a cold wind, for example, may stimulate nonpainful or painful sensations which are perceived in the lost leg.

The Diabetic Who Thought His Foot Was Still There
Joe Downy, a sixty-one-year-old man with diabetes mellitus and hypertension that had first been recognized when he was in his thirties, had his right foot amputated because of ulcers and severe pain around two of his toes. He survived the surgery well, but after the anesthesia wore off he felt severe pain in his stump and phantom foot. This was

a constant throbbing that involved his whole nonexistent foot from the ankle to the toes. It felt as if the whole foot below the ankle was in a vise. Added to this, he had frequent unpredictable paroxysms of lancinating pain lasting a few seconds and radiating downward into the phantom toes, which felt as if they were being bitten by a giant crab.

A variety of pain medications were tried postoperatively without success, including intravenous morphine he controlled himself. He was taken to the operating room for an indwelling epidural catheter to deliver a potent opioid, fentanyl, as well as a local anesthetic. Gradually the pain lessened with treatment and all pain medications were discontinued. This was not the end of it, though. The pain reappeared soon afterward and has continued to come and go for many years, even affecting the upper leg. A variety of drugs have been used, as well as electrical nerve stimulation (TENS) and spinal-cord stimulation, none of which provide sufficient relief.

Treatment for Phantom-Limb Pain

Treatments vary according to the severity of the pain and the degree of a person's incapacitation. The first order is to take care of relatively easily correctable sources of pain, like ill-fitting prosthetics and decreased blood supply in the stump. Acupuncture, biofeedback training, and supportive measures such as relaxation and stress-reduction techniques are sometimes helpful; and physiotherapy and psychotherapy can be as important as drugs or surgery, which rarely afford long-lasting relief.

Medications. As with other types of neuropathic pain, anticonvulsant drugs such as Tegretol are frequently prescribed, and tricyclic antidepressants such as Pamelor and other drugs such as Mexitil may help. Narcotic analgesics may be useful when someone has severe chronic phantom pain.

Transcutaneous electrical nerve stimulation (TENS) is effective for short-term treatment, but its effect diminishes with time. It is interesting that some studies have found that when TENS is applied to the healthy limb, opposite the amputated one, it was shown to decrease or totally eliminate the phantom-limb pain. It was thought that the stimulation from TENS stimulated nerve fibers that modulated or inhibited pain pathways involving the phantom limb.

Sympathectomy, which involves cutting or otherwise destroying the sympathetic nerves supplying the stump of the amputated limb, may be performed in people who respond well to repeated local anesthetic blocks without lasting effects. However, long-term results here are predictably disappointing.

Other surgeries disrupt the connections between the peripheral nerves, the spinal cord, and the brain. There are a number of procedures: DREZ lesion destroys the dorsal-root entry zone to the spinal cord and has a reported 60 percent relief of pain, although long-term results are not good.

Spinal-cord and deep-brain stimulation, when it works, doesn't usually last. It also may not address the problematic pain-producing abnormal brain circuitry. Theoretically, *cortical stimulation,* or stimulation of the covering of the brain, may help control phantom pain by stimulating the cortical areas no longer receiving normal input from the amputated limb. This stimulation, if used early enough, may diminish the tendency of the brain to form abnormal, potentially pain-producing circuits, while limiting the abnormal firing of pain-processing neurons that used to process painful stimuli from the amputated limb.

Smoke and mirrors. A new technique that sounds like a magician's trick may also help the condition. A recent study from the Center for Brain and Cognition at the University of California suggests that we can learn to regain control over the parts of the brain that cause phantom sensations and pain. By looking at his or her remaining, opposite limb using a system of mirrors to create an optical illusion, the patient can see the mirror image of the remaining limb. The mirror image coincides visually with the phantom feeling from the former limb. By watching the movement of the real limb superimposed over the area of the missing limb, phantom-limb pain may be resolved.

Prevention

It may be possible to prevent phantom-limb pain by paying careful attention to preoperative pain relief. In some amputations, chronic pain and inflammation in the limb prior to amputation may sensitize the central nervous system. A few years ago, a technique called preemptive analgesia was touted as a means of preventing sensitization and phantom pain. In this technique, the anesthesiologist uses continuous epidural injections of local anesthetic and narcotic for at least two to three days before surgery. In theory, the epidural anesthesia serves to block the sensitizing pain input of the peripheral nerves from the diseased and presumably painful limb to be amputated—before the limb

is actually removed. Preemptive analgesia may be particularly important in amputating chronically painful limbs, such as those of people
affected by advanced atherosclerosis (including diabetics) or malignant tumors—situations in which phantom pain is most likely to develop. Preemptive analgesia has received mixed support in academic
studies.

Phantom pain underscores the baffling complexity of the nervous
system and the extraordinary, poorly understood relationship between
the mind and the body. The physician or medical scientist grappling
with phantom pain walks up to the enormous problem, looking up in
awe and amazement, glimpsing the glorious intricacy of the nervous
system. And then, contemplating a treatment for a painful malfunction of the system, we trip and fall flat on our faces, skinning our noses
and chins on the sidewalk of therapeutic defeat. Much more work has
to be done to understand, prevent, and treat the fascinating but often
horrible phenomenon called phantom pain.

Other Treatment for Neuropathic Pain

Spinal-cord stimulation (SCS), which may be viewed as a form of
TENS (see chapter 2), is used to treat pain from damaged nerves,
spinal roots, and CRPS, and to treat the painful and destructive side
effects of atherosclerosis, or clogging of the arteries, in the legs. Spinal-
cord stimulation may relieve about 50 percent of pain in 75 percent of
patients who meet strict selection criteria.

In a hospital operating room or special X-ray room, using local
anesthesia and light sedation, little electrodes are implanted under the
skin with the stimulating ends placed in the epidural space over the
spinal cord. Electrodes are placed either in the neck to control arm
pain, or in the lower thoracic region to control leg pain. These electrodes are attached to an external stimulator, which stimulates the
electrodes and thereby the underlying spinal cord. You feel some tingling in the bodily areas supplied by nerves from the stimulated cord.
The electrodes are positioned by trial and error until the tingling covers the area of pain. This may take up to an hour, during which time
you are awake, working with the doctor to guide the placement of
these electrodes. Once the wires are secured, you spend a few days in
the hospital while the stimulator parameters are fine-tuned for the best
response. A small battery-powered stimulator and the connecting
wires can be surgically implanted under the skin like a pacemaker.

Stimulating the cortex is an exciting pain-relieving procedure evolving in neurosurgery. The cortex, or covering of the brain, contains the neurons that process information about our environment and govern much of our activity, including our perception and reaction to pain. By stimulating small areas of the cortex, we can control otherwise untreatable neuropathic pain. Because this procedure is reversible, it is unlikely to cause lasting side effects. Technically, this procedure is similar to spinal-cord stimulation. In this case, electrodes are implanted over the brain after careful stimulation of the brain in the operating room, and wires from the electrodes are connected to a small stimulator, usually implanted under the skin. This technique shows great promise. It may be particularly effective in helping people like Mr. Stoneblood who suffer from pain following brachial plexus avulsion. It may also be helpful with other forms of neuropathic pain, including phantom-limb pain.

Exciting new drugs, such as the potent venom of certain poisonous Pacific sea snails, are being evaluated. In the wild the venom immobilizes curious fish that get too close. We may be able to use this venom in treating chronic pain, including neuropathic pain. A synthetic form of the venom has been shown to inhibit pain transmission by blocking the release of neurotransmitters in pain pathways of the spinal cord. Unfortunately, the venom cannot be given by mouth or intravenously, as it will be broken down and thus become ineffective. It can be injected into the spine where it can act locally with few side effects.

KEY POINTS
About Neuropathic Pain

- Neuropathic pain is nerve pain that has its source either in or outside the nervous system.

- This kind of pain can occur for no diskernible reason and go away the same way.

- The pain can be extremely frustrating to diagnose and treat.

- If untreated, this pain can worsen and spread and become less treatable.

- Pain in a limb that is no longer there is very real pain.

8

Prevention and Treatment of Painful Sports Injuries

Take calculated risks.
This is much different from being rash.

—GEORGE PATTON

Everyone has become a weekend warrior, and as the growing list of patients in sports-medicine clinics will attest, many are getting hurt. Some of these warriors fail to warm up to their sport with stretching or training and sprain or strain some part of their body. Others may fail to wear shin guards on the soccer field and sustain injury, or use improper technique in swinging a golf club and pull a muscle.

Many sports injuries, such as getting hit in the head with a hardball, cause acute pain, which, after treatment, usually goes away. However, there are many causes of chronic pain that come from the playing fields, such as torn ligaments from jumping or pivoting, nerve damage from racket sports or cycling, or spinal-cord injury from a fall. Notice how everybody cheers when the fallen player, who has just been beaned with a hardball at eighty-five miles an hour, bravely gets up and goes back into the game. Is this heroic or foolish? Failure to evaluate and treat what may appear to be a minor injury often leads to chronic pain and other disabilities.

The emerging field of sports medicine is bringing more attention to conditions such as tennis elbow, jumper's knee, runner's heel, and the football player's migraine. Even carpal-tunnel syndrome, the wrist condition that we equate with long hours of working at a computer keyboard, was originally known as cyclist's palsy or handlebar palsy because of the number of bikers who contracted the condition.

Your tennis elbow is the same as the tendinitis the factory worker gets from lifting parts off an assembly line. It makes little difference whether it is Monica Seles or Jane Doe who suffers the injury. The only difference between the two injuries is that the professional may feel greater emotional stress because the injury might be professionally disabling, so she may have a greater need for more complete and comprehensive rehabilitation. Thus, she may go directly to a sports-medicine specialist.

SPRAINS AND STRAINS

Most sports injuries are simple contusions, otherwise known as bruises, that result from a direct but blunt trauma to a soft tissue, including skin; muscle; tendons, which connect muscle to bone; and ligaments, which connect bone to bone. Such injuries occur when you are hit with that fastball or pass the volleyball with your wrist instead of your fist. Contusions cause pain, swelling, and bruising on the surface of the skin. The pain from contusions varies according to the severity of the injury.

Sprains and strains are often confused. Strictly speaking, a sprain is an acute traumatic injury to a ligament, and a strain is an acute traumatic injury to the muscle–tendon junction.

When a knee is extended beyond its normal range of motion, for example, or an ankle is forced into a position it does not normally achieve, the joint becomes dislocated or incompletely dislocated (a condition called subluxation). Almost any significant sprain involves some actual or partial dislocation. Treating a sprain means treating the injured ligament.

Strains, on the other hand, are commonly called *pulls*. A strain is a forceful but indirect injury to an area of muscle and tendon. This means that a strain usually develops through overuse or misuse, not from a blow or cut. Football, skating, and martial arts are often responsible for strains.

Joints are precise and well-honed connections between two or more bones. Ligaments stabilize the joint in conjunction with the muscles, and prevent abnormal movements of the joint. The main symptom of damage to a ligament is pain that is usually sharp and localized in the actual area of the sprain. There may be an audible pop or snap at the time of injury. Swelling and limitation of movement occurs to various degrees, depending on the severity of the injury. Severe sprains are characterized by a sense of instability, which athletes refer to as a sensation of looseness.

The secondary effects of injury to a ligament are often more troublesome than the original injury. Swelling and spasms of the muscle can limit motion and the normal use of the joint, and when muscles and ligaments are not used, they can become unstable. The most severe sprains are characterized by a total loss of integrity of the ligament—that is, there may be a complete tear. (Later we'll get to the most well-known ligament injury, in the knee.)

The most important part of the physical examination will be to determine whether there is abnormal instability of the joint. For severe sprains, correct diagnosis requires X rays and other diagnostic tests, especially MRI.

In terms of treatment, the best first aid for a sprain involves rest, ice, compression, and elevation (RICE). Nonsteroidal anti-inflammatory drugs can be taken to relieve the pain. If there is no instability, the physician may prescribe short-term steroids. Surgical repair of the injury requires the expertise of an orthopedic surgeon.

Most people think that strains are always a consequence of overstretching a muscle, but they occur more often during forceful muscle action when the tension is abruptly and actively increased. This could happen to someone who has not played golf for a long time and then, without warming up, swings at the ball with enough force to whack it all the way to the next tee.

Strains can also develop when a muscle is forced to perform a task beyond its capabilities, causing it to tighten up and become weaker. Most athletes practice stretching and flexibility training to avoid pulling any muscles.

Strains can occur in the tendon, in the muscle, or at the junction of the two. Some tearing-type fractures are also considered strains. These are called avulsion fractures and they occur when a tendon and its bony attachment pull loose from the surrounding bone. Such fractures can be tiny and barely visible (like most cases of tennis elbow), or they can be large, as when hamstring muscles are affected. Injuries to the hamstring, the long muscle in the back of the thigh, occur most often among sprinters, hurdlers, and high jumpers. These injuries often recur and become chronic.

The major symptoms of a strain are pain when stretching the involved muscle and muscle spasms (tightening up). If the strain is more severe, the symptoms are abrupt and immediately disabling, often accompanied by an audible snap or pop that can be heard by others. After the initial burst of pain, symptoms of these severe strains can subside, making these injuries sometimes initially less painful than minor strains.

Bruises may appear on the skin a few days after a strain because of broken blood vessels releasing blood into the tissues. The extent of swelling, if any, usually parallels the severity of the strain. When hamstring muscles are ruptured, for example, the swelling can be substantial; less swelling usually accompanies tennis elbow. The limitation of motion caused by the strain also varies according to the severity of the injury.

Like the treatment of sprains, the initial treatment of strains is aimed at preventing bleeding and swelling. When there is an incomplete tear, it is important also to try to lessen any potential long-term disability associated with muscle spasm.

As with sprains, initial first aid in the form of RICE (relative rest, ice, compression, and elevation) should begin as soon as possible. If the muscle or tendon ruptures, the limb should be splinted. The physician may recommend performing X rays or MRI to help judge the severity of the strain or avulsion fracture. Exercises and strengthening programs can help restore lost range of motion.

OVERUSE INJURIES

Sports-medicine specialists consider overuse injuries the most pervasive type, with the possible exception of impact injuries that occur in football or hockey. Because overuse injuries are not immediately disabling, as acute traumatic injuries can be, they are easily overlooked. Left untreated, they can become well established and more difficult to treat.

Some common overuse injuries of the muscles and tendons include tendinitis, myositis, myotendinitis, and tenosynovitis. Tendinitis means inflammation of a tendon. Myositis refers to an inflammation of the muscle, myotendinitis to inflammation of both the muscle and the tendons, and tenosynovitis to inflammation of the tendon sheath or covering. As you can see by these names, any or all of the muscle-tendon unit can be injured.

Tendons get inflamed with overuse and can swell up and cause problems in the heel, shoulder, and other areas. *Achilles' heel* did not become a metaphor for a person's weak spot for no reason. Achilles tendinitis is one of the most frequent types of sports tendinitis. It usually results from too much of an unaccustomed activity such as running up hills or repetitive jumping. It also can develop if you change the height of the heel on your running shoe.

Rotator-cuff tendinitis is the scourge of baseball pitchers. Four important muscles in the area of the shoulder and shoulder blade, or scapula, are affected. The shoulder is a ball-and-socket joint and the cuff is just what it sounds like, a cuff around the socket. Rotator-cuff injuries occur mainly during throwing sports, but can also happen to a skier who falls over on an outstretched arm.

Bicipital tendinitis, or tendinitis of the biceps, is relatively uncommon and also occurs predominantly in people who participate in throwing sports but who are in poor condition.

Peroneal tendinitis refers to inflammation of the peroneal tendon of the calf. It results from forceful bending forward, as when a skier falls forward over a ski. This tendinitis occurs infrequently, but it usually requires surgery.

Overuse injuries similar to so-called pitcher's elbow and Little Leaguer's elbow are also common in other sports, such as golfing, gymnastics, tennis, wrestling, and weight lifting. Even sensitive violinists develop a similar kind of painful elbow.

An abrupt increase in running up hills or sprinting causes a condition called plantar fasciitis. Both of these actions require you to push off with your toes, which puts the soles of the feet in jeopardy. Plantar fasciitis involves either partial or complete rupture of the plantar fascia, which is the fibrous sheet covering the muscles in the sole of the foot.

Iliotibial-band syndrome causes irritation and inflammation on the outer side of the knee and is a well-recognized cause of the knee pain that often affects runners. In one study of more than one thousand distance runners, iliotibial-band syndrome accounted for some 5 percent of all cases of lower-limb musculoskeletal complaints. This kind of knee pain has also been reported among sprinters and participants in racket sports, not to mention aerobic dancers and cyclists.

Stress Fractures

Stress fractures can occur in nearly every bone of the body and are exceedingly common in both sports and industry. They are essentially failures of the bone to adapt to increased demands. Stress fractures occur when forces that are applied to the bone exceed the strength of the bone, deforming it until a microfracture occurs. The stress could result from a repetitive small load or weight bearing on the bone, causing an overuse injury, such as occurs when a runner increases mileage on a weekly basis. When a figure skater tries to learn a new jump, this adds a very large load to the bone.

Common sites of stress fractures are:

- the shaft of the tibia (shinbone) in basketball players, runners, and ballet dancers, which accounts for about half of all stress fractures seen in athletes

- the humerus (in the upper arm) from throwing, pole vaulting, and racket sports

- the ulna (inner bone of the forearm) from racket sports, volleyball, and drumming, and in offensive linemen

- the pelvis in runners

- the lumbar spine in gymnasts, dancers, weight lifters, and football linemen

- the big toe in sprinters, fencers, and rugby players

Women are especially vulnerable to stress fractures when they are in what is known as "the athletic triad." This is a combination of excessive athletic activity, weight loss, and menstrual abnormalities. With continued excessive exercise and excessive weight loss, the estrogen level drops, causing menstruation to stop and leading to bone loss.

Pain is often the only symptom of a stress fracture; early in the course of the injury this may be an aching sensation or just weakness or cramping. If swelling occurs, it is usually late in the course of the injury. Tenderness, like swelling, may be present, but only if the involved bone is in a location where it can be easily felt, such as the ankle.

Stress fractures are difficult to see on X rays. CAT scans provide a better means of diagnosis. Treatment involves stopping or modifying the activity that produced the stress fracture. A rule of thumb is that before gradually returning to the activity that caused the stress fracture, you must be absolutely pain-free for ten consecutive days.

Anterior Cruciate Ligament (ACL) Injuries

Notice how many basketball players wear knee braces because they either have or don't want to have a torn ACL. Most sports fans have seen at least one basketball player crumple to the floor after coming down from a jump shot and twisting a knee, as WNBA center Rebecca Lobo did forty seconds into the 1999 season, which kept her out of the game for the rest of the season.

Injury to the knee is possibly the most common sports injury to a joint. Knee injuries may be acute or result from overuse, together accounting for about 15 percent of all sports injuries. Anterior cruciate ligament (ACL) injuries represent a large portion of these knee injuries, most often occurring while playing basketball, soccer, or volleyball.

The ACL is one of four ligaments controlling and safeguarding the kneebone (patella). The knee is a hinge joint held together by these four ligaments. The two collateral ligaments straddle the knee on either side. The other two ligaments are situated deep inside the knee, crossing each other: these are the anterior cruciate ligament (toward the front of the knee) and the posterior cruciate ligament (toward the back of the knee). Both cruciate ligaments are attached to the end of the thighbone (femur) on one side and to the top of the shinbone (tibia) on the other side.

The ACL supports the knee, keeps it stable, and controls how far forward the shinbone slides relative to the thighbone. A certain amount of motion or sliding is normal and necessary for the knee to function, but too much motion can damage other structures in the knee and lead to chronic problems. This crucial ligament, which keeps the knee balanced when you walk or jump, is one of the most common causes of chronic pain in sports.

The most common injury is a complete or partial tear of the ACL. A tearing injury can happen if you come to a quick stop while running and change direction at the same time. A tear could also develop after pivoting, landing from a jump, or overextending the knee in either direction.

Other sports-related injuries to the ACL include dislocations (sprains) and injuries from stretching the ligament away from the bone (strains).

An audible pop or snap usually accompanies an ACL injury. The degree of pain varies, but it can be severe. Swelling usually occurs within six hours, but the extent of the swelling can be reduced if ice is applied and/or the knee is splinted.

Women are at least three times more vulnerable to ACL injuries than men—some trainers and team doctors claim the ratio is as high as five to one. There are several theories to explain this discrepancy but no sure answer yet. Some say that women have a narrower knee structure, that they land in a more upright position after they jump, or that they rely more on their quadriceps than their hamstrings. We don't know the answer yet, because women have only relatively recently begun to get involved in sports in great numbers.

At any rate, exercises for both men and women can help develop the muscles that support the bones and ligaments of the knee, which reduces the chance of serious injury. For a correct diagnosis if you do get injured, be sure to explain the anecdotal history of the injury to the doctor who examines you. The doctor will try to determine the amount of motion that exists and the extent of a tear, if any, and may manipulate the joint in what is called Lachman's test.

Other structures, such as the cartilage and other knee ligaments, could also be injured, therefore other tests may be performed to see whether the injury is limited to the ACL. X rays can detect a fracture. Sometimes an MRI of the knee also may be necessary to evaluate the cartilage and determine the best treatment.

Ice is usually applied at the time of injury to reduce swelling. Modifying the amount and type of physical activity and wearing a hinged sports brace is standard treatment until the knee is healed. The goal of physical therapy is to strengthen the muscles around the knee to compensate for the injured ligament.

Surgery may restore stability and protect the cartilage of the knee from being damaged, particularly the meniscus cartilage, which serves as a shock absorber between the ends of the bones. If the meniscus is damaged too badly, arthritis could result.

In general, surgery is recommended for young people who frequently perform sports that involve pivoting, as well as for people who have injury to other parts of the knee in addition to an ACL tear.

There are a number of different types of surgery that are used to repair or restore the ACL. If there is a tear, the orthopedic surgeon may prefer to perform a graft, using another tendon from around the knee to surgically replace or reconstruct the injured ACL. This can be either an autograft (from a person's own body) or an allograft (from another person's body).

While the hospital stay is usually overnight, with intravenous pain medication and antibiotics, rehabilitation may take six to nine months of physical therapy.

SPINAL INJURIES

Football has received the most attention as a cause of acute spinal injuries, but surprisingly, most injuries to the spine occur during water sports such as high diving. Other sports implicated in severe spinal injuries include downhill skiing, wrestling, gymnastics, rugby, ice hockey, and horseback riding. The most well known of such accidents happened to the actor Christopher Reeve, an experienced horseman who was thrown from his mount and broke his neck. He was left paralyzed from the neck down but has led a remarkable life in helping others like him and raising money for more medical research into spinal-cord injuries.

Injuries of the spine can be catastrophic if they are not given proper care. It is not unusual for someone with a fractured neck to walk fairly well after the injury and appear relatively unharmed for a period of time. If these traumatic fractures are ignored and not X-rayed or treated by immobilization, there can be serious neurological and other consequences. When in doubt, the neck or, less commonly, the thoracic spine should be stabilized to protect the spinal cord until full evaluation can be made.

Usually, if enough bone is broken and ligaments are torn to disturb the spine, there is significant local pain, providing the impetus for a full evaluation following stabilization.

Herniated disks caused by sports activity usually call for only some restriction of activity along with anti-inflammatory medications, oral steroids, narcotics, and possibly epidural steroid injections. Physical therapy is important to decrease the pain and to improve the mobility and strength of the back and muscles of the lower extremities.

See chapter 6 for a detailed description of low-back pain, its treatment, and how the pain is referred and felt in various regions of the body.

Spondylolysis: A Type of Vertebral Fracture

Spondylolysis is a condition unique to the lumbar spine in which a fracture occurs in the component of the vertebra that connects the facet to the rest of the vertebra. Spondylolysis may represent the late consequences of a stress fracture or it may be simply a birth defect. In the worst case, this condition may lead to spondylolysthesis, or slippage of one vertebral body over another. In this condition, part of a vertebral body breaks (a process called lysis) and the spine may become unstable, with one vertebra shifting over another (a process called lithesis), and this instability may cause ensuing pain. If there is enough slippage of one vertebra over another, the spinal canal and the foramina become smaller, the cauda equina and the roots in the foramina can become compressed, and leg pain, weakness, and numbness may ensue. Fortunately, many cases of lysis heal without evolving to lithesis.

If spondylolysis is caused by an injury, it is more than likely caused by repetitive stress of the lumbar spine, as may occur in football, dancing, gymnastics, and weight training. In fact, spondylolysis is the most common cause of low-back pain in football players. Such pain is usually localized on one side.

Conservative treatment for spondylolysis is rest, application of ice, and giving up the pain-producing activity for several weeks to months. X rays, bone scans, and CAT imaging can confirm or rule out a stress fracture, which is reversible if detected early enough. If your symptoms do not respond to conservative treatment or if you have spondylolisthesis, you need a neurosurgeon or orthopedic spine specialist. This condition may ultimately require fusion surgery to restabilize the spine. Always get more than one opinion before agreeing to such a major procedure. Read chapter 6 for a thorough explanation of spinal-fusion surgery.

INJURIES TO NERVES

Nerve damage can result from many sports. For example, carpal-tunnel syndrome is a neuropathy of the wrist common to cyclists and racket-sports athletes. Neuropathic-pain-producing sports injuries include injuries caused by entrapment, compression, or trauma.

Neuropathies

In cyclists, the pudendal nerves in the genital area or the sciatic nerves may be injured from the pressure (compression) of the bicycle seat, resulting in pain or tingling in the genitalia of men or down the leg of cyclists of either sex. Adjusting the seat or getting a larger seat with more padding can help relieve symptoms due to compression of these nerves.

One entrapment neuropathy that affects cyclists involves the median nerve within the carpal tunnel. The carpal tunnel is a narrow, bony channel through which the median nerve passes on the underside of the wrist. Prolonged bending of the wrist can irritate the median nerve within this tunnel, causing nerve inflammation, with resultant pain, tingling, and even weakness of grasp involving the thumb and the first three fingers. Adjusting the angle of the handlebars and wearing padded gloves can help relieve symptoms of compression of the median nerve in the carpal tunnel.

Other nerves vulnerable to injury are:

- the axillary nerve of the shoulder, from throwing or swinging a racket

- the radial nerve of the arm, also from throwing or swinging a racket

- the long thoracic nerve, on the side of the chest wall, below the armpit, from weight training or swimming the backstroke

- the suprascapular nerve, above the shoulder blade, from fencing or pitching a baseball

- the femoral nerve of the leg, from gymnastics

As with other injuries, rest is the foremost factor in healing. Chapter 7 covers various treatments for the relief of neuropathic pain.

Sciatica

True sciatica is irritation or inflammation of the sciatic nerve or the spinal roots supplying this nerve. Cyclists, weight lifters, and rowers are at risk because of repeated straightening of the forward-bent spine against pressure. This results in excessive pressure on the lumbar disks. The most common cause of sciatica is a bulging or herniated lumbar disk. The major symptom of sciatica is pain all along the sciatic nerve from the buttock down the leg into the foot. There also may be low-back pain or neurological and sensory symptoms, such as numbness or abnormal sensation, including tingling.

The athlete often first seeks medical attention after an episode of severe low-back pain and sciatica, which may be on one or both sides, correlating with the disk herniation. The acute pain is caused or increased by coughing or sneezing.

Refer back to chapter 6 for treatment for sciatica. As with other injuries of this kind, treatment may include rest, physical therapy, and the use of analgesics.

Burners and Stingers

Burners and stingers sound like something you'd find at an Irish pub. In fact, they are injuries that occur when the nerves of the neck and shoulder area become stretched by forcible depression of the shoulder, such as when blocking or tackling on the football field using the shoulder as the primary point of contact. The network of nerves emanating from the lower cervical and the first thoracic spinal roots, known as the brachial plexus, controls the sensation and movement of the arm and shoulder. Burners and stingers are so named because of the burning or prickling pain of the upper limb that characteristically follows a block or tackle. They are the most frequent nerve injuries to football players.

Symptoms of brachial-plexus injuries can be confused, and coexist, with spinal-cord injuries, the latter of which can also cause burning upper-limb pain. Injury to the brachial plexus may result in a feeling of weakness without pain. Stingers can recur, so the best advice is to refrain from contact sports until the symptoms are gone and muscle strength is restored.

Most frequently people with these symptoms are X-rayed or referred for electromyography (EMG) to determine the extent and type of injury. The major treatment, as with other injuries to the neck and spine, is time and rest.

HEADACHES

Heading a soccer ball with the front of your head contracts various neck muscles. Doing this repeatedly seems a pretty obvious way to get a headache. "Footballer's migraine" was first reported in British athletes participating in soccer games (in most of the world, football refers to what Americans call soccer). It was described as a classic migraine that occurs immediately after the player hits the ball with the frontal region of his head.

Headaches can result from a host of sports or exercise traumas, including neck trauma and concussions (see chapter 4). Another type of headache is associated with weight lifting and occurs when pressure is increased in the chest while lifting, which, in turn, causes the veins of the neck and head to dilate, causing increased pressure within the skull. These headaches cause abrupt, burning pain, gradually persisting as a dull steady ache around the back of the head or neck. Scuba divers experience migrainelike headaches from changes in air pressure. Mountain climbers have altitude headaches and marathoners experience effort headaches. But the most common type of exercise-induced headaches that occur in athletes are tension headaches.

Tension headaches occur as often in athletes as in the general population; in both cases, they are at least partly related to fatigue, anxiety, depression, and emotional stress. Pain from tension headaches is dull, constant, bandlike pressure in the back of the neck and head and radiating to the forehead and temples. Tension headaches may strike every day or they may happen only seasonally. They vary in intensity, location, and duration.

Traditional treatment for tension headaches includes nonsteroidal anti-inflammatory drugs (NSAIDs) and Tylenol (acetaminophen). To reduce the stress that may be provoking or compounding the headache pain, psychotherapy, hypnosis, and biofeedback are sometimes included in treatment of persistent headaches.

Other adjuvant therapies include neck massage, hydrotherapy, dosing with Tylenol or NSAIDs prior to sports activity, and iontophoresis (the use of electricity to drive certain medications through the skin). Sometimes anti-anxiety or antidepressant drugs are given, particularly if there is a psychological component to the tension headache. See chapter 4 for a further description of other types of headaches and headache remedies.

BASIC PREVENTION AND TREATMENT

The treatment of sports injuries, naturally, depends on the type and severity of the injury. There are simple first-aid measures to institute as soon as any injury that requires medical attention occurs. For example, if you should fall in your yard when playing touch football, your goal is to prevent the swelling or bleeding that follows any rupture of the blood vessels, causing a bruise. Swelling and bleeding distort normal anatomical relationships, resulting in pain and loss of motion. For acute injuries, try to stop the bleeding and swelling with RICE (rest, ice, compression, and elevation). Then seek medical help, preferably from someone who specializes in sports medicine or orthopedics, to be sure that splinting or surgical repair is instituted when needed.

See a specialist in orthopedics or sports medicine if you have a severely painful injury or limitation of movement, because you may have a fracture or a severe sprain. In either case, the injured limb may need to be immobilized with a splint.

As soon as any swelling has subsided, you should begin range-of-motion and strengthening exercises. An orthopedic surgeon or specialist in sports injuries can suggest the types of exercises to do, and help you get started.

Most sports injuries are not life-threatening, but there are enough exceptions that cost lives or lead to extreme disability that you should bone up on your sports first aid.

There are four important rules to follow in the event of a serious, life-threatening injury, which are also essential for less severe injuries.

• Control bleeding.

• Prevent further injury.

• Restore blood flow to the injured part.

• Stabilize and repair broken bones, including the spine.

Preventing further injury generally means to properly pad and splint the injured limb before an injured person is allowed to move. "Splint 'em as they lie" is the rule most emergency-medicine caregivers follow. Virtually anything that provides some stability can be used as a splint, including adjacent body parts, rolled blankets, clothing, or pillows. Rigid or semirigid splints with some padding generally provide the best immobilization of a limb.

Participating in sports means our bodies are active and getting a good workout that keeps us healthy. But it's always better to be safe than sorry, so train properly, use good equipment, and learn how to use your body so you don't hurt it. Chapter 2 offers some good advice about avoiding injury.

If you have been injured, consider changes you can make to avoid more such injuries, such as a different bicycle seat or more suitable running shoes. The last resort, of course, is to try a different sport.

Sports massage, strength training, warming up, and cooling down should always be part of your regime in any sport.

KEY POINTS
About Painful Sports Injuries

- Most sports-related injuries are from overuse.

- Contusions and most sprains and strains should be treated with RICE (rest, ice, compression, and elevation) as soon as possible to prevent further pain.

- Failure to adequately warm up by stretching muscles is the cause of many painful strains and sprains, as well as nerve damage.

- The bones, muscles, tendons, ligaments, nerves, and spine are most vulnerable to sports injury.

- When sports injuries are not properly treated, they can become chronic and painful.

9

Gynecologic Pain

*Man endures pain as an undeserved punishment:
woman accepts it as a natural inheritance.*

—ANONYMOUS

Gynecologic pain is actually one of the most poorly understood and managed types of pain. Until recently, the primarily male medical and research establishment spent very little time and money studying what they called "female problems." For example, a senior gynecologist colleague admitted that he used to consider the pain of PMS (premenstrual syndrome) purely psychological and thus could offer no treatment to his patients. He knows, now, that the pain and other symptoms of PMS are real and that there are sound medical treatments for them.

If pain emanates from the pelvic region or the perineum (between the anus and the vulva), a woman in pain will usually first see a gynecologist, internist, or urologist. She may then be referred to a surgeon or even a psychiatrist. Such women usually visit a pain clinic only if the pain has been chronic for some time and all other treatments have failed. In my practice, I rarely see patients with gynecologic pain unless it is related to cancer pain.

Remember what you learned in chapter 1 about test-negative and referred pain? Pelvic pain is a good example of referred pain, in which pain from one organ is readily felt as coming from another area. This phenomenon is particularly relevant in the pelvic area because of the way nerves and their receptors are distributed throughout this region. The internal or functioning parts of the pelvic organs generally do not contain pain receptors, while the walls of the membranes lining the abdominal and pelvic walls (peritoneum) do have a rich supply of nerves. Therefore pain impulses that might emanate from a visceral organ get caught up in a kind of overflow of impulses, and the origin of the pain is apt to be poorly localized by the patient and often perceived at a surface site far removed from its actual source. For example, pain from the uterus is most commonly felt as lower-abdominal pain and pain from the cervix as coming from the lower back or sacrum. Pelvic pain can also be of gastrointestinal or urological origin.

Because women with many painful gynecologic conditions also may have bladder and bowel disorders, this suggests that there may be a common causal link among some disorders of the pelvic organs. Nonetheless, most of these conditions have no known specific cause and therefore treatment is often what is called empirical—that is, the doctor will treat on the basis of analogy and experience, without full knowledge of the actual cause of the disease.

Up to 20 percent of women with chronic pelvic pain are not given a clear diagnosis or reason for their pain. Physicians have labeled the pelvic problems they understand poorly as "CPPWOP" (chronic pelvic pain without obvious pathology). The ambiguous name of this syndrome speaks volumes. It is also striking that the syndrome, which has been known since the early part of the nineteenth century, has been given many different names over time, such as "syndrome of pelvic congestion and fibrosis," "pelvic sympathetic syndrome," and "pelvic neurodystonia." The names imply vastly divergent causes, demonstrating a basic lack of understanding. For example, *fibrosis* refers to the formation of tissue with a fibrous structure, one of which is scar tissue, due to obvious injury or ongoing inflammation. *Neurodystonia* refers to a disorder of increased muscle tone, thought to be due to abnormal nervous-system activity.

The main unifying element of CPPWOP is that it is *pain with the characteristics of pain of gynecologic origin and with no known cause (gynecologic or otherwise) or visible evidence of a disease process.* CPPWOP is a test-negative condition. Thus, it is no wonder that women who complain of pelvic pain frequently find themselves going from doctor to doctor, including psychiatrists. In fact, many women with difficult-to-treat pelvic or genital conditions such as vulvodynia (chronic pain of the vulva), interstitial cystitis, and dyspareunia (painful intercourse) are frequently referred to a psychotherapist. If a woman cannot be diagnosed as having endometriosis or cancer, or some other condition in which there is a visible mass or other sign, many physicians will not believe her pain is real. Instead of considering that the depression and anxiety a woman may be experiencing might be the *result* of the test-negative painful condition, gynecologists often think of the mood changes as the *cause* of the gynecologic pain.

The remaining 80 percent of patients with pelvic pain have conditions that are generally easier to diagnose and quite often easier to treat.

Other known gynecologic conditions that can cause a type of recurrent but not chronic pelvic pain are dysmenorrhea (severe and prolonged cramping just before or during menstruation), mittelschmerz (intermenstrual pain), and premenstrual syndrome (PMS). Pelvic adhesions are another cause of pelvic pain, but are usually a postoperative complication or a consequence of disorders such as pelvic inflammatory disease or endometriosis (see pages 176–79).

RECURRENT PELVIC PAIN

Dysmenorrhea and mittelschmerz are usually experienced as aching and cramping just before or during menstruation and briefly during ovulation. If cramping pain occurs along with a feeling of abdominal pressure and minor bleeding, and if the patient could possibly be pregnant, a physician would need to rule out an ectopic pregnancy or miscarriage before any treatment. If the menstrual cramps are severe and worsen during the last few days of a woman's menstrual flow, she may have endometriosis (see page 176). Persistent dysmenorrhea also may be a symptom of fibroid tumors. PMS has diverse physical symptoms, ranging from water retention and bloating to backaches and headaches, and a range of psychological symptoms including irritability and depression.

These recurrent types of pelvic pain are usually easily treated with over-the-counter medications and sometimes lifestyle changes. For example, over-the-counter NSAIDs like aspirin and Advil (ibuprofen) often ease the pain because of their antiprostaglandin properties. When the pain persists, stronger medications may be required.

Lifestyle changes can help, such as reducing salt intake and eating nutritionally balanced meals, especially foods high in calcium. Hot baths and heating pads can also relieve symptoms. Regular exercise increases the circulation and helps carry off excess body fluids in the form of perspiration. Exercise also stimulates the brain to release endorphins, the body's natural narcoticlike or opioid painkillers.

Chronic Pelvic Pain

Chronic pelvic pain may indicate endometriosis, pelvic inflammatory disease (PID), displacement of the uterus, or cancer. It may also be caused by posterior parametritis, an inflammation of a portion of the uterus above the cervix.

Endometriosis

Endometriosis is a benign but painful condition in which cells from the endometrium (the lining of the uterus) become scattered outside of the uterus, most commonly on or within the ovaries. Ordinarily, excess endometrial tissue is expelled as part of the normal menstrual cycle. When for some reason endometrial tissues spread outside the endometrium, they may scatter to distant regions such as the appendix, vagina, bladder, lymph nodes, lungs, eyes, and even the brain, much in the same way that tumors spread. Endometriosis may cause not only physical pain but also infertility, with its attendant depression, anxiety, and frustration.

The cause of endometriosis is unknown, although it most often occurs in women twenty-five to forty-five years of age and responds to the cyclic rise and fall of ovarian hormones. Pregnancy protects against endometriosis because of the changing levels of hormones during this time. Women who develop endometriosis are often well educated and prone to high stress. This has led to the stereotypical characterization of endometriosis as a career woman's disease occurring largely in women who have delayed marriage and childbearing to pursue a career. In truth, endometriosis also occurs in very young women. About 15 to 20 percent of women with endometriosis have a positive family history of the disease and up to 40 percent of women who develop endometriosis are infertile.

It is estimated that seven to eight million women in the United States suffer from this condition, although only 10 to 15 percent of cases are diagnosed. According to a 1991 article in the *American Journal of*

Obstetrics and Gynecology, the incidence of endometriosis may be as high as 51 percent in women seeking evaluation of pelvic pain.

Symptoms of endometriosis include generalized pelvic pain and menstrual disturbances, including dysmenorrhea. Menstrual pain usually worsens during the last few days of the period, but over time, the pain begins ever earlier in the cycle. When the pain occurs prior to menstruation it is often misdiagnosed as pelvic inflammatory disease (PID), a tilted uterus, or polycystic ovaries. An internal pelvic examination will reveal an irregular pelvic mass lying behind the uterus or on the ovaries. This mass becomes more tender when progesterone and estrogen levels rise prior to menstruation. It also can cause painful bowel movements.

Painful intercourse is usually the symptom that drives a woman with endometriosis to seek a physician. Other symptoms of endometriosis might include gastrointestinal complaints from rectal deposits of endometrial cells or urinary-tract symptoms if the bladder is affected. A few women develop what is called an acute abdomen when a single noncancerous mass that contains endometrial tissue (called endometrioma) ruptures. An acute abdomen requires surgical evaluation to determine the source of the problem and rectify it. The extent of the disease is usually not comparable to the extent of the symptoms. Women with severe disease may have mild symptoms while those with minimal disease may experience great diskomfort.

Treatment varies according to a woman's age, the extent of her disease, and whether or not she would like to have a child.

Self-care measures to relieve the pain include the use of a heating pad or hot water bottle applied to the lower abdomen. Aspirin, Tylenol, or Advil also may help relieve pain. Cutting down on caffeine may also help because it seems to aggravate the pain in some women. Tampons may contribute to menstrual cramping, so some physicians recommend using sanitary napkins instead. Women with endometriosis also may have a tipped uterus, which makes intercourse painful. The use of a natural lubricant and trying new positions that allow for penetration without pain may help.

For women who still want to become pregnant and whose symptoms do not respond to self-help measures, hormone therapy may be prescribed temporarily to stop ovulation and induce a pseudopregnancy state that enables the abnormal tissue to shrink. Endometriosis naturally goes into remission during pregnancy and after menopause.

The use of continuous high doses of oral contraceptives is another treatment, although these drugs cause weight gain and potentially serious side effects, including the possibility of a blood clot in the legs, lungs, or elsewhere. Recently the U.S. Food and Drug Administration approved the steroidal drug Danocrine (danazol), which induces a kind of pseudomenopause by directly preventing the surge of one hormone at midcycle. The only FDA-approved drug for the treatment of this condition, Danocrine is a form of the male hormone testosterone. There are some side effects, such as weight gain and swelling, but these are reversible. Long-term use, however, could lead to more complicated side effects such as a deepening voice and an increase in body hair.

Other medical treatments that have been used to relieve the pain of endometriosis include progesterone, androgenic (malelike) steroids, and drugs such as Lupron that suppress the production of female hormones by the body. These therapies may bring relief of the symptoms, but the symptoms often return once the drug is discontinued.

The only treatment that offers a complete cure is the surgical removal of the involved tissues. Surgery also may be necessary to determine whether the lump behind the uterus is endometriosis and not cancer. In advanced cases, a total hysterectomy may be required, along with removal of the ovaries and fallopian tubes (salpingo-oophorectomy). Whether or not a woman chooses this surgery depends upon whether or not she wants to have children.

Pelvic Inflammatory Disease (PID)

Pelvic inflammatory disease (PID) is the term used to describe any extensive infection in a woman's pelvic organs: the uterus, fallopian tubes, ovaries, and surrounding tissues. If untreated, these infections can result in sterility and even become life-threatening. Symptoms and signs of PID include pain and tenderness in the lower abdomen, painful intercourse, heavy vaginal discharge, unusually early or heavy menstrual periods, and irregular bleeding between periods. When acute, PID may also cause fever and backaches.

PID is often caused by a vaginal infection with a strain of the chlamydia bacteria, a sexually transmitted infection that goes untreated and spreads throughout the reproductive tract. PID also may be caused by streptococcus or staphylococcus bacteria contracted during the insertion of an intrauterine device or after a pregnancy or abortion.

Symptoms of PID are easily confused with endometriosis, a functional ovarian cyst, mittelschmerz, or a urologic or gastrointestinal problem that results in pelvic pain. The best way to avoid this confusion is with a laparoscopy, an endoscopic diagnostic test in which the pelvic area is viewed through a tube inserted through a tiny incision just below the navel.

The best treatment for PID is a ten-day course of antibiotics at the first signs of infection, bed rest, and abstinence from intercourse.

Fibroids

Fibroids (also called leiomyomas) are benign tumors that grow in the wall of the uterus and have a fibrous structure. Their cause is unknown, but various hormones, such as estrogen and growth hormone, appear to play some role in their development. These are the most common types of tumors that affect the female reproductive organs, occurring in about 20 percent of women over thirty. They range in size from microscopic to the size of a grapefruit and usually grow in clusters. The fibroids grow more rapidly when the body has ample estrogen, as seen, for example, in women taking birth-control pills or during postmenopausal hormone replacement.

Fibroids usually grow very slowly and rarely cause pain, but they can, so they are included here. The most common symptoms of fibroid tumors include heavy menstrual periods and infertility. When pain is present it is usually described as a feeling of heaviness and pressure in the lower abdomen. If a woman experiences sudden, sharp abdominal pain, this could indicate that the fibroid has become twisted and lost its blood supply. When this happens, emergency surgery is usually necessary.

Fibroids usually do not call for treatment, except when periods are overly heavy. Iron supplements may be needed because excessive blood loss may cause anemia. Laser surgery through the vagina may be used to remove these tumors in some cases; otherwise they are removed using more conventional surgery, approaching the tumors from the lower abdomen.

Functional Ovarian Cysts

Functional ovarian cysts are related to normal cyclic ovarian function and occur during the reproductive period. In most women these cysts resolve spontaneously during the next menstrual cycle and cause no problems. Sharp and sudden pain may arise if the cysts rupture or become twisted during physical or sexual activity. The pain might arise suddenly and resolve within hours, or it could result in an acute abdomen, requiring surgery (laparotomy). Sometimes the symptoms of functional ovarian cysts are similar to those of an ectopic pregnancy: pain on one side, delayed periods, and a mass that can be detected on physical examination. Because of this, doctors always rule out an ectopic pregnancy before further treatment.

Episodic one-sided pain that eventually becomes constant and localized may indicate that torsion (twisting of the cysts) has occurred. In these cases surgery will most often be required—either a laparotomy to remove the cysts or surgical removal of the affected ovary.

Interstitial Cystitis

Interstitial cystitis is not a gynecologic condition, although its major symptom is pelvic pain. It is a chronic urologic disorder of the bladder with no known cause. Because various antimicrobial drugs have been used with little success, interstitial cystitis is probably not caused by a microbe. Other theories hold that interstitial cystitis stems from the body's immune system attacking the bladder, or suggest an allergic reaction. This cystitis also has been considered a neurological disorder.

Symptoms include pain, usually around the pubic area; painful intercourse; and urinary urgency and frequency without any obvious infection. The pain is classically related to bladder filling and is relieved by voiding, although some people also experience pain after urinating. The typical patient sees three to five physicians before getting the correct diagnosis.

Because the underlying cause of interstitial cystitis is unknown, clinicians have tried a wide range of therapies. Foremost among these is a procedure called hydraulic bladder distention, which is performed under a light general anesthetic.

Various medications are used to relieve the pain, including the tricyclic antidepressants. Another drug that has recently been approved by the FDA to treat interstitial cystitis, and which appears to have a somewhat mixed effect, is sodium pentosan polysulfate (Elmiron). Other drugs currently under study include an antihistamine and the calcium channel blocker, nifedipine (known as Procardia), which lowers blood pressure. Both are intended to control the activity of cells involved with the allergic response.

When all of these measures fail, drugs such as dimethylsulfoxide are injected into the bladder itself. Dimethylsulfoxide (DMSO) acts as an anti-inflammatory, analgesic, and anesthetic agent. DMSO may be combined with other drugs, such as sodium bicarbonate, steroids, and heparin, all in the hope of decreasing the inflammation of the bladder. This treatment is usually repeated weekly over a period of six to eight weeks. Another drug used the same way is the topical antiseptic Clorpactin (sodium oxychlorosene), but it is painful and must be administered with an anesthetic.

Still other treatments that have been used for patients with this form of cystitis include transcutaneous electrical stimulation (TENS; see chapter 2) and electrocautery or lasers to excise ulcers. Surgery is performed as a last resort, and often produces no benefit.

Vulvar Pain Syndrome

Chronic pain of the external genitalia is usually difficult to treat because of the overlap between this and other anatomic locations in the pelvic and perineal areas and the referral of pain from one area to another as a result of the close relationship of the nerves that supply the area.

The vulva is the external female genitals, including the vaginal orifice, the labia majora and minora, the pubic area (mons pubis), and the glands surrounding the vagina (vestibular glands). In 1983, the Seventh Congress for the International Society for the Study of Vulvar Disease defined *vulvodynia* as chronic vulva discomfort characterized by burning, stinging, irritation, and rawness.

Another condition related to vulvodynia is called vulvar vestibulitis. The same congress defined this condition as a syndrome of severe pain when the vestibular regions are touched or during attempted vaginal intercourse. These and other disorders known as vaginismus and burning vulvar syndrome share a number of symptoms and therefore are better characterized under the catchall term *vulvar pain syndrome.*

As many as 15 percent of the women seen by gynecologists may have vulvar pain syndrome and it is particularly common among white women in their forties who have not had children. Women with vulvar pain syndrome have a high incidence of allergies and infections with human papillomavirus candida. They often have a history of sexual abuse as well.

As with many of the gynecologic disorders, the cause of vulvar pain syndrome is unclear. Some of the theories that have been suggested include infections, allergies, or reactions in which the body attacks itself, or a psychological basis. Although it has not been proven, some investigators claim that vulvar pain syndrome may be caused by a fungal infection such as candida. Under this premise, many women are treated with topical antifungal agents without a culture having been taken. Chronic pain of the vulva also may be caused by postherpetic neuralgia (see chapter 7) or Sjogren disease (a disorder in which the body attacks itself), which may cause dryness and irritability of the vulval mucosa, or mucous-covered skin.

Treatments range from sitz baths, antibiotics, antifungals, and anti-inflammatory agents to steroid creams and lubricating agents, with little success. Topical anesthetic creams have been used to allow intercourse. Injection of a substance called interferon alpha, designed to alter the body's immune response and fight viruses and tumors into inflamed vulval areas, also has had varying success.

Other Causes of External Genital Pain

Pruritus vulvae is the sensation of itching in the vulva, which may be severe enough to be considered pain. The most common causes of vulval itching are candida and trichomoniasis, but there may be other causes. Treatment is usually directed at the cause, presuming it can be established.

Most cases of severe painful itching are treated by gynecologists. However, when it becomes chronic and severe and all else fails, these patients are occasionally referred to pain clinics.

Dyspareunia refers to painful sexual intercourse. There are many possible causes, including psychological ones, particularly during the first attempt at intercourse. Dyspareunia is different from vaginismus, or failure to allow penetration because of involuntary muscle spasm, although pain may be experienced at the same time. Vaginismus may have a psychological basis or may be caused by local disorders of the vulva and vagina. Any discomfort during intercourse can be accentuated by a lack of lubrication. An anesthetic block around the cervix may temporarily help the symptoms, but management is directed mainly at excluding anatomical or infectious problems and exploring any possible underlying psychological manifestations. Medication designed to expel excess body water; hormones; or psychiatric drugs may help. A program of exercise to strengthen the muscles and increase abdominal muscle tone, such as Kegel exercises, is also helpful. Kegels involve alternately contracting and relaxing the muscles of the perineal area, which can help relax the muscles and relieve pelvic pain. Biofeedback can be successful if you can isolate the pelvic floor and contract and relax these muscles appropriately. The most commonly used technique to monitor biofeedback involves measurements of pelvic-floor activity through a vaginal probe, both when you are at rest and during a contraction. Acupuncture is another technique that has been used to treat pelvic pain. For more information on some of these techniques, see chapter 2.

KEY POINTS
About Gynecologic Pain

- Until fairly recently, much gynecologic pain was often dismissed as being of psychological origin because very little solid scientific research had been done.

- This type of pain is often test-negative and is also misdiagnosed because the pain may be referred from nearby organs in the pelvic area, such as the gastrointestinal or urinary system.

- Failure to correctly diagnose and treat gynecological pain can lead to more serious conditions, including infertility and widespread cancer.

- Gynecological pain often is either recurrent or chronic.

10

Reducing the
Pain of Cancer

In war nothing is impossible, provided you use audacity.
—GEORGE PATTON

Imagine an orchestra of broken instruments playing as loudly as possible. The tuba wheezes, the drum thuds, the violin snaps, and the horn flies off into the audience just as a fire alarm sounds backstage. This cacophony of sounds, this collision of mishaps, is like the insistent pain of cancer. It is a din of damage from confused sources, all of which clamor for attention.

Cancer pain is the most feared of all pain because it implies a serious and often life-threatening disease. Yet my goal here is to demonstrate that cancer pain, in its purely physical form, is a mixture of musculoskeletal, neuropathic, and visceral pain, and can be well controlled in the vast majority of patients. I cannot assuage fears about dying and death. But I can inform patients that dying in pain, or wanting to die due to unrelieved pain, is not only unnecessary but unacceptable in our society today. Cancer pain can and should be controlled.

Cancer is a term for a number of diseases that involve unchecked multiplication of cells, creating malignant tumors in the organs (intestines, lungs, stomach, ovaries, brain, and so on) or tissues (muscle, bone, skin). Cancer cells may travel—that is, metastasize—from the primary tumor through the blood vessels or lymph channels to other sites in the body and form new, secondary tumors or metastases. Cancer invades surrounding tissues and may block passageways. For example, cancerous tumors of the digestive system may obstruct the passage of food in the stomach or waste matter in the colon, causing dilatation of the colon, pain, and potential perforation of the distended bowels and life-threatening infection. Cancerous tumors destroy tissue such as bones, resulting in painful fractures, and damage nerves, causing neuropathic pain, weakness, numbness, and possible problems urinating or defecating, which can also be painful. Much of the pain from cancer is a sign that a tumor is damaging something.

Some 20 to 50 percent of cancer patients are in some pain at the time of their diagnosis, and 55 to 95 percent experience pain at advanced stages. In one study, moderate to severe pain was present in 50 percent of cancer-pain patients, and another 30 percent had excruciating pain.

People are more afraid of the pain of cancer than they are of the cancer itself. Yet, by the late 1980s, a review of the treatment of 1,229 cancer patients in Milan, Italy, showed that the pain of 891, or 70.9 percent, had been successfully relieved by oral narcotics. Today, in 75 to 85 percent of cancer patients, pain can be adequately controlled through narcotics and other pain relievers given noninvasively—orally, rectally, or in skin patches. Up to 20 percent of cancer patients whose pain is not relieved by noninvasive drug delivery will obtain relief with intravenous or subcutaneous narcotics. On average, only 10 percent of cancer patients or fewer may require extraordinary, high-tech means of pain control, such as injecting narcotics into the spinal canal or, when all else fails, by destroying nerves carrying pain impulses from the body to the spinal cord or brain. Thankfully, these high-tech interventions are often quite helpful. For this small group of patients, the high-tech world that brought us the rat race becomes a savior. If patients knew all this, one of the great clouds of fear facing human beings in this country and around the world would lift. Informed patients could and would demand pain relief, and with enough persistence, they would always get it.

Increased pain in a cancer patient usually, but not always, means the cancer is growing. Often, the best pain control for growing tumors is to get them to stop growing, using radiation, chemotherapy, surgery, and sometimes other means of locally controlling the tumor, such as injecting toxic materials directly into it. Along the same lines, radiofrequency energy, converted to heat and delivered through electrodes inserted into the tumor, has been used to destroy some noncancerous bone tumors and damage cancerous liver tumors without damaging surrounding tissue. Cancer pain is highly variable in terms of its source and location, involving the musculoskeletal system, the internal organs, and the nerves, often all at the same time, and frequently in different parts of the body. More than 60 percent of cancer patients have pain as a direct result of a tumor invading surrounding tissue. Common pain-inducing cancers include breast and lung cancer.

Since different types of pain respond best to different medications, most cancer patients need several different kinds of pain relievers during their treatment, given in various ways, as well as pain-relieving anticancer treatment such as irradiation of pain-causing tumors.

Cancer treatment itself causes pain. In one study, slightly over one-quarter of patients had pain due to cancer therapy—surgery, chemotherapy, and radiation.

Patients also experience pain that is unrelated to cancer, such as the pain of arthritis that flares or continues even as the cancer becomes the center of the patient's and the doctor's concern. Approximately 10 percent or fewer of cancer patients have pain unrelated to cancer or its treatment—myofascial pain, diabetic neuropathy, osteoporotic fractures, and spinal stenosis, for example. Cancer usually strikes older people, who are subject to more sources of pain. Sometimes the pain of other conditions such as osteoporosis or arthritis masks or conceals the pain of a cancerous tumor that has developed.

Conversely, people sometimes fear their pain indicates cancer when it has another source. When a man who is told his prostate cancer is in remission wakes up with terrible pain in his shoulder, he fears that his cancer is back and has metastasized. However, he is just as likely to be experiencing the pain of arthritis, so he should not make his own diagnosis.

Proper tests and radiological studies will support the doctor in evaluating the condition. Remember, any new pain that persists for several weeks without a known cause calls for a high-quality physical examination by an experienced physician as well as high-quality diagnostic MRIs or CAT scans, supplemented by X rays, bone scans, and other tests as needed. New pain in any patient with a history of cancer should be considered a possible recurrence of the cancer until proven otherwise.

An oncologist or pain specialist experienced in treating cancer patients must diagnose the source, or sources, of pain in order to treat them most effectively. Pain due to new or progressive cancer must be treated, not just with pain medication, but with anticancer treatment directed against the malignant tumor causing the pain. Conceptually, this is no different from giving painkillers to reduce pain while preparing a patient for setting a broken bone or for surgery to remove a large disk herniation causing sciatic pain and disability. Pain treatment should occur in conjunction with treatment of the disease.

Determining the cause of the pain is particularly important because anticancer treatment—not just painkillers—should be used whenever possible to control pain and dysfunction resulting from progressive or recurrent cancer. The objective here is to control the pain by controlling the source of the pain. Along with pain medication, surgery, radiation, and chemotherapy should always be considered as means of helping to control cancer-related pain, even when these therapies cannot cure the underlying cancer.

PAIN FOLLOWING SURGERY

Cancer surgery can be terribly effective in helping to treat—and at times cure—patients. Indeed, if tumors are found early enough, they can be cured by surgery alone, because they never spread. Unfortunately, if cancer is a three-act play, we walk into it all too often in the second act—too late for surgery alone, or possibly anything else, to achieve a cure. However, surgery can help preserve function and relieve pain from spreading tumors that wrap around bowels or the spine, or that invade the brain, for example.

Every time you have an operation, nerves are pulled, pushed, and cut, usually with no long-term ill effect. Certain body areas are more likely to cause significant postoperative pain, some of it permanent. This kind of pain is usually due to nerve damage or scarring, and some people may be more likely to experience such scar formation than others.

Lung-cancer surgery (thoracotomy), in which the ribs are divided along the side of the chest, can cause prolonged pain along and around the incision. It may last for years. The pain is constant and is accompanied by tingling or burning within the area of the scar; the surrounding skin will be supersensitive and sometimes numb. Typically, the pain is made worse with movement, even breathing. The nerves running under the ribs are particularly sensitive to trauma. Post-thoracotomy pain can be seen after chest surgery other than cancer surgery. However, in the cancer patient, pain is never just pain until proven otherwise. Thus the hullabaloo when this kind of pain exists following surgery for a malignant lung tumor.

Chronic postoperative pain may occur after radical or simple mastectomy, or even lumpectomy, for similar reasons. However, radical mastectomy is the biggest offender, causing chronic pain about 5 percent of the time. Pain usually begins one to two months following the surgery because of damage to a branch of a particular nerve supplying the skin. Here again, the nerves run under the ribs, in this case, the first and second ribs.

The pain is tight and burning in the back of the arm or the armpit and it spreads to the front of the chest. Moving makes it worse, and many patients hold their arms to their sides with the elbow bent. Pain following mastectomy may result in a painful "frozen" shoulder. To get this shoulder moving, it is usually effective to prescribe a two-week course of oral steroids, or local injections of lidocaine and steroids into and around the shoulder, followed by physical therapy.

Pain following mastectomy must be differentiated from radiation-induced scarring of the nerves going into the arm (many patients receive radiation to the area after a mastectomy) or a tumor invading the nerves that enter the arm just near the armpit. This is not always easy. Fortunately, mastectomies are far less common now, given the advances in managing breast cancer.

Extensive neck surgery for control of cancer may lead to constant burning pain in an area of diminished sensation on the skin of the neck. Painful tingling sensations and electric-shock-like pain may exist as well. This pain comes from the damage of various nerves supplying the skin of the neck.

Following removal of a kidney (nephrectomy), some patients develop painful tingling sensations combined with a sensation of numbness, heaviness, or fullness over the back near the surgical scar, just below the ribs, and in the lower front abdomen and groin. This is because of damage to the first lumbar nerve, which exits the spine below the level of the ribs. In cancer patients, a tumor growing near the spine, under the incision, should be considered.

Amputation may be part of the treatment of a sarcoma—a malignant tumor arising in a bone, such as one of the bones of a leg. Even without cancer, this type of surgery often results in prolonged postoperative pain and other sensations. Nearly all amputees experience phantom-limb sensations (see chapter 7).

All of these postoperative pain problems usually require medication for neuropathic pain, possibly some narcotics, or TENS (see chapter 2). Injection of local anesthetics and steroids into painful scars may give some relief, although I have never been very impressed by the long-term benefits of such interventions. Interventional procedures to control the pain also include destroying the pain-carrying nerves, permanently or at least for several months. Indwelling tubes placed in the spine or, in the case of chest pain, in the chest cavity can deliver pain-relieving medication continuously. Some neurosurgical procedures may be used with good results as well. Those are covered in chapter 7.

RADIATION THERAPY

Radiation is a highly effective and necessary therapy for controlling or even curing cancer. It is highly effective in treating cancer pain of all types. This includes pain from tumors in the bone, internal organs, and nerves. Radiation therapy aimed at painful tumor-ridden bone relieves pain in 70 to 80 percent of patients within a few weeks. Patients with pain due to bone metastases from breast, lung, and prostate cancer make up about 20 percent of referrals to radiation-therapy departments. Therapy can be performed in a short or long course, depending on the patient. A short course of radiation can relieve pain in twenty-four hours but has more long-term side effects than a longer course.

Another form of radiation helpful in treating bone pain due to metastatic cancer—particularly from prostate cancer—is supplied with radioactive isotope, strontium[89], injected intravenously. It is incorporated into bones, like fluoride. Radioactive strontium[89] kills certain tumors in bones and relieves pain. However, it takes three to four weeks to work and may damage the blood-cell-forming marrow, limiting severely the ability to receive future chemotherapy—which also often attacks the marrow. Therefore, strontium[89] is usually given as a last resort.

During the nuclear tests of the 1950s and '60s, a sister isotope of strontium fell to the ground, was ingested by grazing cows, and ended up in milk, scaring everyone and prompting the beginning of the test-ban treaties. Radiation can cause damage to anything (skin, organs, bones, blood vessels, and nerves) in or around its path. The damage may be temporary or permanent. A sunburn-type effect is an example of temporary radiation skin damage. Unfortunately, radiation scarring of nerves often causes *permanent* delayed pain, and even later weakness, numbness, and other dysfunction. Radiation can also cause nervous-system tumors to grow, four to twenty years after the radiation was delivered. This is un-like chemotherapy-related damage, which often diminishes with time.

Nevertheless, radiation can be used with fewer untoward side ef-fects than ever before, thanks to improved diagnostic radiological de-vices (MRIs, high-quality CAT scans) that help us to better see exactly where tumors are, as well as better techniques of focusing and deliv-ering therapeutic radiation. However rarely, radiation still damages nervous tissue—probably causing problems in less than 5 percent of patients. I recently saw a fellow physician as a patient. He had devel-oped throat cancer and was cured by surgery and radiation. However, the radiation damaged his spinal cord, lying in the spine behind his throat, leaving him with disabling pain from his neck down. His pain is neuropathic in quality and difficult to control. It and the side effects of his medication—not the cancer itself, which was cured—caused him to leave work. Radiation-induced pain can be as bad as cancer pain.

Occasionally, when we irradiate tumors in the throat, other parts of the neck, or the chest (usually for lung cancer), it can deleteriously af-fect the spinal cord. Irradiating the spine itself—usually to treat metastatic tumors or nearby lung tumors in the back of the chest, or bones affected by myeloma (a blood and marrow cancer)—will also involve radiating the cord running within the spine and rarely causes cord damage. Irradiating a lung tumor just behind the collarbone or the armpit following breast cancer can damage the nerves in the neck going into the arm. Irradiating the back of the pelvis (behind the hips) or the back of the lower abdominal area (around the spine under the ribs) can result in damage to the nerves going into the legs. Gyneco-logic, urologic, and colon cancers; metastases to bones in this area; and tumors arising in the bones of the pelvis may all be irradiated, and some patients may develop radiation damage to the peripheral nerves in the back of the pelvis or even the cauda equina.

Unfortunately, the frequent alternative diagnosis to radiation-in-duced pain is residual or recurrent cancer, or radiation-induced scar-ring mixed with tumor. Remember what I said about pain in cancer: it is usually not a good thing. It usually—admittedly, not always—sig-nals a tumor. Trying to distinguish a tumor from radiation scarring is difficult. At times the most sophisticated MRIs and other tests can't tell. Sometimes even a surgical biopsy is inconclusive. This diagnosis is especially difficult early on in the growth of the tumor, when tumor cells may be irritating nearby nerves without yet having grown into an easily defined mass. Ultimately, time provides the diagnosis—the tumor either declares itself or doesn't. If the tumor recurs, it must be treated with anticancer therapy. If there is not a recurrent tumor, pain medication must be continued—in some cases indefinitely.

CHEMOTHERAPY

Chemotherapy is a useful means for controlling or even curing breast cancer, Hodgkin's disease, and other similar cancers of the lymph system, some leukemia, and testicular cancer. Even when chemotherapy can't cure, it can extend survival and control tumor-related pain by shrinking tumors. Most chemotherapy has side effects, such as nausea and hair loss, which are not painful and can be controlled with medication or which resolve with time (hair grows back).

However, some chemotherapy can cause pain. While usually short-lived, it can be quite annoying and needs to be treated. For example, many anticancer drugs cause transient painful sores (like canker sores) in the mouth following their administration. Some drugs also cause transient abdominal and other pains.

Some very important, potentially lifesaving drugs cause several short-lived but potentially troublesome pains. Neupogen is used to build up the patient's infection-fighting white-blood-cell count when cancer or its treatment has lowered the number of white cells. By giving the patient Neupogen, higher doses of potentially curative chemotherapy can be administered with less risk of killing patients with the infections that are side effects of the chemotherapy. Yet Neupogen causes transient moderate bone pain in about one-quarter of those receiving it. This pain is usually not so severe as to require narcotics. It also causes mouth sores, which may need treatment.

Unfortunately, most chemotherapy is given in repetitive cycles of a few weeks, at least for several months. Moreover, some effects of chemotherapy may be cumulative—they become worse with more treatment over time.

Other chemotherapy-related pain lingers and may worsen with more treatment. Most of the long-term painful side effects of chemotherapy result from peripheral neuropathy, damage to the peripheral nerves that supply the arms and legs (see chapter 7). Fortunately, most of these neuropathies are not severely painful; they are more often annoying constant tingling sensations, coupled with a sense of numbness. Only occasionally do they become quite disabling and painful.

Cisplatinum is a drug that can cause a neuropathy, with loss of sensation, weakness, or pain, usually in the legs or arms. This drug and its relatives are often used to treat testicular, bladder, ovarian, lung, head, and neck cancer. The drug is discontinued if neuropathy becomes a severe problem. However, the neuropathy usually improves with time.

Vincristine and similar compounds—like the more modern Navelbine—may similarly cause a neuropathy, usually affecting the feet and hands. These drugs may also cause all sorts of transient aches and pains, occasionally severe. Many of these drugs are used in treating Hodgkin's disease and other lymphomas, and some cases of breast and lung cancer. Drugs such as Vincristine are often given until a patient has enough neuropathy that it becomes difficult to button a shirt, for example. Once that point is reached, the drugs are often withheld.

For years I treated one patient with a residual painful neuropathy from a Vincristine-like drug, which had been used to help cure his Hodgkin's disease. He is a plumber who stands for up to six hours per day, often carrying heavy loads, and wears metal-toed shoes to protect his feet from inadvertently dropped pipes. He has chronically painful, slightly numb feet, and cannot move his toes well.

I prescribed four Percoset (a moderately strong narcotic mixed with Tylenol) daily several years ago and it has been very helpful in reducing his pain. I doubt his neuropathy will improve further, but he is quite alive, without cancer, earns a good living, and has raised a wonderful family over the last twelve years.

Some drugs cause transient as well as persistent painful side effects. Taxol causes transient mouth sores and muscle and joint aches. The former may require treatment and the latter, though usually mild, may be severe at times, requiring narcotics. In the long term, Taxol may produce mild and, rarely, severe neuropathy, which may result in disability and pain. Reducing the dose helps control severely painful side effects. The drug is used to treat lung, breast, and ovarian cancer, as well as Kaposi's sarcoma.

TREATMENT WITH CORTICOSTEROIDS

Corticosteroids are used to shrink certain kinds of cancerous tumors, such as lymphoma. As noted in chapter 3, they also have potent anti-inflammatory properties, they shrink swollen tissues, and they significantly reduce pain due to bones, spinal roots, or peripheral nerves damaged by tumors. Quite amazingly, they also restore function to nervous tissue compressed or invaded by tumors, which becomes swollen and produces various neurological deficits, depending on the structure involved. Compression of nerve roots and peripheral nerves may produce pain, weakness, numbness, or bowel and bladder dysfunction. A damaged spinal cord may cause any of the above symptoms except pain. Similarly, a brain tumor may result in sleepiness or even coma, confusion, problems speaking and seeing, as well as weakness or numbness. The treatment of cancer may damage the tumor, causing it to swell temporarily as it dies. This side effect of successful anticancer therapy may further compress surrounding nervous tissue, worsening pain and neurological function.

Steroids, given by mouth or in high doses intravenously, combat these negative effects of swollen nervous tissue. They may be given in a short course or, if the tumor cannot be eradicated, for months. However, they weaken the strength of certain bones, due to accelerated osteoporosis, and more quickly, may result in destruction of the upper portion of the leg bone, which connects the leg to the hip joint. If this weight-bearing joint is destroyed, severe to excruciating pain may occur. The pain may be controlled with narcotics and NSAIDs.

Ideally, a damaged joint should be replaced with an artificial joint or else the patient may not be able to move an otherwise painful hip. This depends on the expected survival of the patient, as successful recovery from joint-replacement surgery requires several weeks of active rehabilitation and follow-up exercises at home.

Another side effect of steroids with prolonged use is that the body becomes habituated to them. When they are withdrawn because they may no longer be needed to control a certain pain, their withdrawal can produce severe diffuse aches and pains in muscles and joints. This is called pseudorheumatism. The only treatment for it is to restart the steroids and reduce the dose slowly—sometimes over several months. In some patients, I have even seen this process take as long as a year.

TREATMENT WITH NARCOTICS AND OTHER DRUGS

Having little or no pain at the expense of becoming a zombie from overly sedating painkillers is totally inappropriate. The majority of cancer patients, for most if not all of their battle with cancer, should be able to think, feel, converse, listen to the news, maintain a physical relationship with their loved ones, and play with their children or grandchildren.

Treatment of pain should enhance, not detract from, the ability to maintain a rich human existence. Oncologists unfamiliar with the pain lexicon often prescribe narcotics in isolation or with Tylenol, instead of more effective drugs. For example, narcotics may be most effective in treating pain in the hollow organs like the stomach or soft tissues such as tendons or ligaments. Narcotics may be somewhat less effective in relieving bone pain, and still less useful in treating neuropathic pain. In one study of tumor-related pain, 21 percent of patients had pain emanating from internal organs, 34 percent had pain from bone metastases, and 45 percent had pain from nerve compression. In other words, the majority of cancer-related pain should be treated with narcotics in combination with other drugs, something many oncologists ignore all too frequently.

Advanced cancer can be treated effectively with various drugs, including narcotics, without causing significant decline in mental function. Unfortunately, while some physicians may know how to choose pain-relieving drugs to use in combination, they may not have the patience or time for the trial-and-error process of selecting the optimal doses, schedules, and method of administration for an individual at a given time in his or her disease. The willingness to try various drugs may be lacking in some patients and families who are worn down by the process of being sick.

Earlier in this chapter, I pointed out that at least 90 percent of cancer patients can get adequate pain relief with skilled use of various kinds of painkillers, including narcotics, given through noninvasive or minimally invasive means that are widely available in the United States (subcutaneous or intravenous delivery). Yet a study of oncologists revealed that 76 percent of those surveyed felt that they insufficiently evaluated patients' pain complaints. Only half believed that they were able to control their patients' pain in a fashion that was "good or very good." About 60 percent of oncologists were reluctant to prescribe enough opioids to control their patients' pain.

When selecting the best medication to reduce pain, the source of the pain should be considered. Pain related to tumor invasion or distortion of internal organs is treated with narcotics as a mainstay of therapy, although other medications may be combined with the narcotics as needed. For musculosketetal pain, which includes bone pain, narcotics should be combined with medications such as NSAIDs or Tylenol. The latter reduce inflammation and related pain associated with tumor invasion. Corticosteroids, which also reduce inflammation and swelling, have been particularly effective in controlling both bone and neuropathic pain due to invasion or compression of nerves by tumor. They also reduce swelling in compressed nervous tissue, helping to restore neurological function.

Both bone pain and dangerous excess calcium in the blood resulting from tremendous bone breakdown can be helped with a drug like Aredia. This is in a class of drugs that prevent bone breakdown. Some of these drugs also are used to fight osteoporosis. Aredia is particularly useful in treating bone-related pain and excess blood calcium associated with breast cancer and a blood-related tumor called myeloma. It may also help control these complications from other cancers such as lung, kidney, and ovarian.

Neuropathic pain, which is more common than bone pain in cancer, is even less responsive than bone pain to narcotics used alone. When necessary, medications for neuropathic pain should be integrated into a multidrug pain-relieving regimen to minimize this difficult-to-treat but all-too-frequent type of cancer pain. Aside from corticosteroids mentioned above, neuropathic pain may be treated with various types of antiseizure medication, certain antidepressants, and certain heart drugs, Mexitil for example (see chapter 7). Unfortunately, oncologists often overlook the best drugs for neuropathic pain.

Some cases of neuropathic pain respond poorly to treatment, or a patient's pain may well be multidimensional, due to damaged organs and bones as well as nerves. In certain patients, high doses of narcotics must be used to diminish their pain. These high doses often cause sedation. One means of combating this side effect is to also use drugs that awaken the patient, such as amphetamines. But these drugs are usually not used by oncologists.

As you can see, some cancer patients who are being treated for their pain by oncologists may be treated incorrectly or in a suboptimal fashion. This is one reason for oncologists to enlist the help of experienced pain specialists in treating cancer pain. On the other hand, patients themselves, or their families, make up another stumbling block to adequate control of cancer pain. As discussed in chapter 3, the general public has the same ill-founded concerns regarding the medical use of narcotics as much of the medical profession. Aside from reluctance to use narcotics, patients often don't even tell their physicians about their pain. In one study, approximately 60 percent of cancer patients did not adequately report pain to their doctors. Some cancer patients feel that discussing the success or failure of their anticancer treatment should be the major topic of conversation with their oncologists. They avoid distracting their doctor with "minor" details regarding their cancer-related pain, even though most cancer patients not on pain therapy have a significant amount of pain. This demonstrates that patients, not just medical personnel, need to be educated about the nature of pain and its treatment.

I usually try quite forcefully to educate and even argue (politely, don't worry) with family members who doubt the need for narcotics in a relative. My usual line of defense is "Tell me *exactly* what your wife or husband is feeling when they try to walk on that bad leg—and I mean *exactly*." I wait a few moments, like a cougar about to pounce on a lamb, waiting for an answer which is never forthcoming. I listen to an uncomfortable attempt to retreat as they ask more questions or describe their relative's pain in a grossly inexact way.

Then I try to point out that the patient's pain is personal and cannot be appreciated fully by anyone else. "Think of the mental pain you have in dealing with your sick relative. That is your own pain, which the other half does not and cannot fully understand. You will never fully understand each other's pain, but you can be sympathetic and compassionate with each other." I stress that by doubting a family member's physical and possible mental pain, you make it more difficult, if not impossible, for them to obtain the most effective and compassionate treatment. This is especially true if they have become invalids and depend on those around them for help in seeking medical treatment. The incredible challenges posed by cancer and the pain it may cause can best be met with a truly supportive family helping the patient.

Severe physical pain usually need narcotics to improve and I discuss with patients and their families the myths of addiction. Next I emphasize that it is my job to decide, with the patient, how best to control the pain using my professional skills. It is exceedingly important to overcome family fears and misapprehensions about using narcotics. Not only will this allow the patient to take narcotics more readily, it will help in overcoming another barrier to adequate narcotic therapy, effectively administered narcotics. Patients become confused about taking tens of pills and often take them incorrectly, with suboptimal pain control and possibly with severe side effects like excessive sedation. Family members may help patients with the logistics of taking their medicine, including recognizing and overcoming side effects.

Finally, when appropriate, I discuss the issue of increasing the need for narcotics over time. Tolerance may play a role in the need for more narcotics over time to achieve pain control (see chapter 3). However, in treating cancer, increased patient need for narcotics is usually a sign of advancing cancer—more pain-inducing tumor. I emphasize that the patients who complain of more pain and demand more painkillers are usually not faking, or trying to get high, or trying to drown out their sorrow about having cancer. They have pain that should be taken seriously.

They should be reevaluated to determine why they have more pain, examined and studied with X rays and other tests. At the same time, they should be treated with higher doses of medication, more effective pain relievers (including more potent narcotics), or possibly a mix of narcotics and other pain relievers given in a fashion that maximizes pain relief while limiting side effects, such as drug delivery directly into the spine. I assure patients and their families that other pain-relieving measures are available, but should be used only if pain can't be controlled well by medication, with acceptable side effects.

The phenomenon of pain-ridden people seeking death with the help of Dr. Jack Kevorkian may be a direct result of this fear of narcotic pain control. The narcotophobes in our society should hang their heads in the same gallows of shame as Dr. Kevorkian. I don't think I have ever met a patient who could not be relieved of a good deal of physical pain by some means or another. I sadly admit, however, that I have met several patients with overwhelming and seemingly intractable psychological and even spiritual pain. I am not sure what to do to ease such terrible suffering. Nor is anyone else I know.

The Polish Woman

During a recent visit to Poland, I met a woman who had tended to her sick father for several years. He had suffered from severe arthritis and a poorly understood chronic abdominal problem. As it turns out, he probably had an undiagnosed, slow-growing colon cancer. Surgery finally diagnosed his tumor, and it was complications from this surgery that eventually killed him, close to three years later. For a while he was in a fair amount of pain, poorly controlled with the medication given to him by his local doctors. Fortunately, his daughter was married to an American who had been bringing her the painkiller Percoset from the United States to help the patient's pain—with excellent pain relief. In her community, for presumed noncancer pain, Percoset or similar medication could not be obtained readily, in sufficient quantities, at any cost. Even when his cancer was finally diagnosed, she still had to supplement the medication his doctors gave him with Percoset in order to adequately control his pain.

How Cancer Affects the Body's Response
to Pain Medication

Treating pain in cancer patients is particularly difficult because cancer or its therapy may permanently or temporarily damage the brain. *A diseased brain is more likely to react poorly to behavior-altering side effects of pain medication.* Cancer more commonly affects people as they age, and the aging process results in some degree of damage to the brain—independent of whatever damage cancer or its treatment causes. This age-related damage may occur even in the absence of senility. Thus, treating the elderly patient suffering from cancer pain is even more difficult than treating young people with cancer.

Cancer and its treatment may also impair the function of both the liver and kidneys, both of which rid the body of drugs. The liver breaks down bodily toxins and medication, and the kidneys eliminate the toxins and medication from the body into the urine. If bodily toxins accumulate, they deleteriously affect the brain, and patients become confused or sleepy—even in the absence of medication side effects.

If medication is not broken down or eliminated, the medication accumulates in an abnormal fashion and the patients become overdosed on an otherwise normal dose of medication. Overdosing from pain medication can result in various problems, depending on the medication—sleepiness, confusion, twitching, staggering, nausea and vomiting, decreased and even ceased breathing (and death). All of this can be prevented and, if necessary, treated, but has to be dealt with on a daily basis by physicians treating cancer pain.

Lesioning Nerves to Relieve Pain

Lesions are deliberate injuries to nerves made in order to block pain impulses from traveling from a painful area of the body through the nerves to the brain. Usually lesions may be made in a minimally invasive manner using radiofrequency electrodes, cryoanalgesia probes, and injected chemicals that destroy nerves. In some cases, open neurosurgical procedures are employed in which nerve fibers are cut (see chapter 6).

You may be one of the small percentage of patients unresponsive to or intolerant of other means of pain control who can benefit from procedures to lessen pain by destroying nerves carrying pain messages. Many, but not all, of these procedures were used more extensively before physicians and scientists developed new pain medications and became proficient at using these drugs in a highly effective manner. Therefore, physicians who can safely and effectively perform some of these less commonly used procedures may not be located near you— you almost always have to go to them. They have specialized X-ray equipment and a trained staff to help them.

Lesions of the spinal cord and brain. The pain-transmitting fibers from the spinal cord up to the thalamus may be lesioned to relieve pain. These neurosurgical lesioning procedures, depending on location and type of pain being treated, have a success rate of 45 percent to more than 90 percent. Pain may recur depending on the procedure. Complications of these procedures include permanent or transient loss of bladder control, weakness, loss of balance, double vision, confusion, painful tingling in the side of the body opposite the lesion, and, in some cases, death.

Cingulumotomy. This procedure doesn't lesion any pain pathways, but lesions a part of the brain involved in emotions. It has been used successfully to treat medically uncontrollable, severe depression and anxiety and to control patients' reaction to pain. Following a successful cingulumotomy, patients are less likely to complain of pain, unless asked. In other words, they may *perceive* pain as they did before the lesion, but *react* to it far less intensely. Some perceive less pain. Fifty to 75 percent of patients who undergo cingulumotomy for pain relief do well at least in the short term. Side effects are similar to those for other brain lesioning procedures.

Chemical hypophysectomy. This involves lesioning the hypothalamus, a structure at the base of the brain that controls hormone function. Alcohol is injected into the hypothalamus using a needle placed through the nose and directed into the base of the skull. This procedure has been performed with good results on cancer patients with pain due to hormonally dependent cancers (breast and prostate) as well as those with other cancers. Pain often recurs in three to four months, and complications do exist, some significant.

Modulatory procedures. Deep brain stimulation involves no lesions but instead employs electrical stimulation of our own naturally occuring opioid-containing centers in the brain. The stimulated centers diminish the flow of pain impulses to the brain from the spinal cord. This procedure is similar to spinal-cord stimulation. Electrodes are implanted in the brain using the help of specialized CAT or MRI scans and are connected to a stimulator, usually implanted under the skin (chapter 7). Patients being stimulated describe such sensations as a glow all over, a feeling of well-being, satisfaction, and pain relief.

Lesioning Procedures Performed Outside the Spinal Cord and Brain

When other means of pain control are unsuccessful, lesions of nerves may be made using injected chemicals, or more rarely, radiofrequency and cryoanalgesia. Patients must be selected carefully for these procedures, which affect pain relief only on a well-circumscribed area of the body. However, for severe pain that is not otherwise controlled, lesioning the nerves transmitting the pain is a reasonable thing to do.

Destructive procedures, especially those involving peripheral nerves, may require some diagnostic nerve blocks. Following appropriate diagnostic blocks, peripheral nerves may be lesioned to control pain in the head and neck, arm, thorax, abdomen, pelvis, the area around the genitals and rectum, and the legs.

Various chemical lesions may be performed to control pain due to cancer (often gastrointestinal, urologic, or gynecologic) invading the nerves of the sacrum. Some of these lesions may result in loss of bowel and bladder control. Different lesions may be performed for the control of pelvic pain with less serious side effects.

Another beneficial pain-relieving block involves destruction of the nerves around the pancreas. This type of procedure is used to control pain in the abdomen and midback from pancreatic cancer, for example. I have performed this procedure on repeated occasions with excellent success and minimal transient side effects. Side effects include some transient decline in blood pressure and pain and long-term destruction of nerves that regulate the rate at which food passes through the bowels. So for a variable period after the procedure patients may have frequent loose stools. Exceedingly rarely the injected chemical may spread back toward the spine and may result in paralysis. I do not know of a patient with this complication.

The covering of the lung cavity can be anesthetized with local anesthetics delivered into that space through a fine, soft catheter or plastic tube. Chemicals used to destroy nerves can be injected into the same space, providing long-term pain relief from tumors invading the chest wall or the organs in the chest.

Other types of pain-relieving injections involve partial destruction of pain fibers entering the spinal cord from a part of the body ridden with tumor and wracked with intractable pain. Controlled injection of liquid lesioning agents into the spinal fluid will result in destruction of certain nerves. These injections are most suited to relieving pain from small areas of the body emanating from muscles, joints, or bones, but not pain from the internal organs or from damaged nerves. These types of injections may result in good to excellent pain relief in 75 percent of patients for an average of two to four months. This should bring about pain relief in a certain area, but may also result in unwanted weakness, numbness, or bowel or bladder difficulties.

All these chemical lesions can be repeated if they wear off.

Radiofrequency lesions of the ganglia of the cranial nerves and spinal roots, and of the peripheral nervous system, may be helpful in controlling well-circumscribed pain from cancer, including focal rib pain, and some tumor-related head and face pain.

Some nerves in the periphery can be partially destroyed using cryoanalgesia, with short-term benefit and little risk.

Vertebroplasty

Vertebroplasty (see chapter 5) is an excellent way to relieve cancer-related bone pain before, during, or after antitumor therapy. This procedure should be considered for patients with severe, focal, bone pain from an invading tumor that is poorly controlled with medication given noninvasively or is controlled with unacceptable side effects. Vertebroplasty should be used instead of "high-tech" pain-relieving measures, such as intraspinal medication, for a localized, excruciating focus in an appropriate injectable bone.

Although it is most often used to treat the vertebrae, vertebroplasty also has been used quite successfully to treat painful metastases to the pelvic side of the hip joint. The cement works best as a vertical brace for bone under compression—like the spine. It will not hold in bones that are horizontal, like the part of the leg that connects to the hip. Vertebroplasty will not restore the height of the spine or straighten it after vertebral body collapse. It should help prevent further collapse and deformity of the spine. The cement, once hardened, strengthens the bone and keeps it from collapsing further. This alone should reduce pain. More than 80 percent of patients treated with vertebroplasty for cancer experience significant, rapid reduction in pain and improved ability to function within a day. The procedure may be repeated if other bones break and become painful.

THE CANCER AND PAIN-MANAGEMENT TEAM

Patients with cancer pain are often treated most effectively with a team approach. This should include adequate analgesic-drug therapy, neurosurgical pain-relieving procedures, nerve blocks, psychological and behavioral therapies, and supportive care. However, a team approach begs the issue of who on the team is responsible for which problem and when. The medical team of pain specialist, oncologist, and others owes it to the patient to answer the following questions long before he or she needs to ask them:

- Which member of the team do I call at 3 A.M. when I need help?

- Which resident is taking instruction from which physician?

- Who is in charge of my care in and out of the hospital?

- Whom do I call when my doctor is away at a conference or on vacation?

Any patient should have answers to these questions, but especially someone suffering from a serious, unpredictable disease like cancer. The more structure built into the patient's life with cancer and the fewer quandaries to be solved at inopportune times, the better.

Oncologists must do their best to cure cancer, but they must also focus on preserving the patient's quality of life afterward. High-quality survival in the incurable patient is equally important. Pain specialists treating cancer patients must make sure that they minimize pain while maximizing alertness, freedom of movement, and side effects of medication.

To treat cancer pain effectively, the physician must understand how different cancers and their tumors spread and cause pain and other disabilities. It's important to understand how the cancer treatment can relieve or cause pain and malfunction of vital organs.

In 1991, the American Pain Society published a list of guidelines for relief of cancer and acute pain. It stated that cancer pain should be recognized and treated promptly and that toward this end, a patient's pain should be noted on his or her chart, along with the methods and success of pain-relief measures. Patient satisfaction should be surveyed, and patients should be told about medications that can relieve pain and promised attentive care for their pain. Doctors and hospitals must define explicitly their policies for advanced pain management, and put systems in place to monitor adherence to the standards.

In today's world of volume-driven managed care, many cancer doctors view these procedures as involving too much work and expense for someone who is dying. Many of these cancer doctors work under a capitation contract. Managed care gives them so much per patient per year, so they don't have an incentive to spend more on expensive pain-relieving procedures. So what happens? Some patients are overmedicated and sleepy, which keeps them quiet. They may not be in pain, but they are not enjoying their last days fully either. Others are undertreated and that is that. Remember, you vote with your feet—what doctors you use; with your pocketbook—how you choose to pay for care; and in the ballot box—for whom you vote. Your medical care is really your choice.

To a brighter future. All of you insist on it and it will happen.

KEY POINTS
About Cancer Pain

- Most cancer pain is underreported (60 percent of patients don't report it) and undertreated.

- Most patients can be relieved of pain with appropriate medications.

- Drugs are one of the most effective palliative treatments.

- Ten percent or less of cancer patients need extraordinary high-tech treatment intervention.

- Up to 85 percent of cancer patients can get good pain relief with combinations of pain medications and narcotics delivered in a noninvasive manner.

- Pain is caused by the cancer, its treatment, and other existing conditions.

- More than 60 percent of cancer pain is caused by a tumor invading tissue.

- Only half of oncologists believe they provide good pain relief.

- At least 60 percent of oncologists are reluctant to prescribe narcotics.

11

How to Get and Pay for the Best Treatment for Pain

BOSWELL: *So, Sir, you laugh at schemes of political improvement?*

JOHNSON: *Why, Sir, most schemes of political improvement are very laughable things.*

—SAMUEL JOHNSON

Nazmija was Bosnian and had immigrated to this country. She came to me with excruciating cramping in one of her legs that had lasted for two years. Ten years before she had had the same problem and a neurosurgeon in Italy, where she was working, surgically treated a disk herniation in her lower back with excellent results. Nazmija had returned to work as a housekeeper and had been pain-free for eight years. One night as she was mopping the floor, she felt the pain shoot down from her back and she said to herself, "It feels like that disk again."

After evaluating Nazmija with MRI, her American doctor saw no anatomical explanation for her pain. He prescribed drugs, but they did not relieve it in the slightest. He then referred her to a pain-management specialist who at first tried more drugs, then decided to implant a pump to deliver morphine into her spine, which was an extraordinary step for extraordinary pain. Even with this "high-tech" method of pain control, she required additional pain pills. Still, she was in so much pain she could not sit down.

Nazmija's son, Gashi, concerned about his mother's painful existence, brought her to see me. She had to lie down on a couch when she came to my office. The MRI she brought me was already two years old and of low quality, yet I was able to detect what appeared to be a recurrent disk herniation involving the same disk that had caused the original problem, diagnosed and treated correctly in Italy. I wanted a better MRI that would give me a fuller picture, but because of the difficulty in performing an MRI with an implanted morphine pump, and the fact that her prior surgery complicated her anatomy, I decided to send her for a CAT scan coupled with a myelogram. Sure enough, these confirmed that she had a small disk herniation in the old location. It had squeezed a nerve root near it, causing her two years of agony.

Nazmija should never have been taking long-term pain medication and should never have had the pump. She should have had surgery. Once she had the disk operation, she was fine, especially when the residual effects of the medication disappeared from her system. Interestingly, the surgeon performing the discectomy noticed that the pump was never properly connected in the first place—another reason she suffered so much for two years.

Through her employer, Nazmija was in a health maintenance organization (HMO) that forced her to get what I felt were substandard MRIs and go to a radiologist who seemed to work more on a volume than a quality basis. He had to review so many films so quickly that he was unable to read them very carefully.

Nonetheless, when I saw the MRI, I thought the problem was a recurrent disk herniation at the same site as before. When Nazmija was bent over mopping the floor and experienced back pain, she recognized her own problem. She was absolutely right, but no doctor listened to her. Instead, they sent her on a painful, very expensive, inappropriate, and relatively ineffective course of treatment. Her case illustrates all the challenges a patient faces in choosing the physician who will help her, and all the challenges that confront a patient in the current atmosphere of medical cost-cutting.

Your doctor's job is to side with you and your pain, to be your advocate to others who don't understand your condition or its treatment. A pain specialist often has to educate patients' families about the nature of severe pain and the appropriateness of using narcotics or other means to treat it. A patient can't get far if the doctor doesn't believe that what you say is important. As soon as I met Nazmija and took her history, I felt certain she had a diagnosable physical reason to have pain. Based on this, I tried to find out what her problem was so she could be treated effectively.

I believe what my patients tell me. Very few have ever caused me to regret doing so. When pain patients are driven to "crazy" states, it is usually because we doctors don't believe them when they say that they are in pain. Often doctors who don't understand something about a patient immediately assume it is the patient's fault. I've done this myself. When I was a student I was sure that a patient was "faking" if he said something was painful to him that I did not think should bother him. I would be angry that here I was trying to take care of people in an emergency room and a "crackpot" was taking up my time.

Recently a woman who came to me for surgery moved around so much during the procedure, despite light intravenous anesthesia, that I could not work effectively. I thought she was anxious, or possibly inattentive. I did not want to give her more anesthestic and I finally asked her if she could try harder to be still. She said she could not because of her diffuse pain from fibromyalgia. What I had thought was a psychological problem was in fact a symptom of a painful disease. The solution was to increase anesthesia, which worked well to diminish the restlessness without causing excessive sleepiness.

A trusting relationship between doctor and patient is essential. The question is which doctor to trust and how to choose one. The inadequate relief of pain is partly due to the fact that people don't "doctor-shop" effectively. Often, people insured with HMOs look in their health-care directory and hope for the best. Some are unaware that they can change medical plans, challenge the system, and become well-informed patients.

Don't expect your medical-insurance company to help you. If you ask one of their clerks where you can find a doctor who specializes in neurosurgery, they will ask you, "What's your zip code?" They assume that nobody wants to go far from home to find a doctor. Consult more knowledgeable sources like doctors you know and professional medical associations, like your state medical society, books like this one, the Internet, and other patients. Ask them what hospitals and doctors have the best reputations for treating your kind of condition.

Once local physicians learn that you are willing to go to great lengths to get help, they may help you interpret some of the information you gather. I see many patients from various parts of the country who have been sent to me by physicians reviewing my Web site at the request of their patients.

Janet came to me from the Midwest, where she was doing sophisticated laboratory work in a highly technological firm. Following a disk surgery several years earlier, she continued to experience such significant back and right-leg pain that she was considering applying for disability. There seemed to be no evidence of anything left in her spine to cause pain from pressure on a nerve root, or evidence that the spine was unstable. She had been to several pain clinics locally without great result, in spite of competent attempts to help her. She was also about to get married and she wanted to begin her married life in a positive state. Janet traveled to New York to see me. I was able to help her through a pain-relieving procedure involving lesioning the nerves from her lower lumbar facets and a ganglion of the lumbar nerve root giving her leg pain. This actually ended all her pain, something I never really expect to happen.

Janet's fiancé paid for the trip and the cost of her care with his credit card. He even took out another credit card to assure that she would have enough money, in the event that that was necessary. He gladly took on debt so that she could get proper treatment. She danced at her wedding six months later and was a very happy bride. They both feel the trip to New York and the financial investment in her care was more than worth it.

Not all patients are so single-minded about getting better—and paying for it out of pocket if needed. Some people are simply unaware they can get better diagnostic tests by spending their own money, beyond what the insurance will cover. Others do not wish to spend anything out of pocket, and, for a serious problem, don't seem to understand the implications of this choice. I don't understand patients with poorly diagnosed conditions, in chronic pain, who say they cannot afford better diagnostic tests, but can sit outside my office, talking at length on a cell phone, planning a vacation that clearly costs much more than the tests *and* various treatment options. Fortunately, I have few such patients in my practice. Like-minded patients and physicians have a way of finding each other.

However, I also know that in today's system, many people are already paying hundreds of dollars a month for health-insurance premiums. People who are self-employed or work for small companies are often uninsured. Many large companies, which traditionally paid for health benefits, are now downsizing and hiring temporary workers so they don't have to pay for health insurance.

Obtaining affordable but high-quality health insurance is particularly difficult for the self-employed or for those in very small organizations. For example, a New York City–based single freelance writer who earns between $40,000 and $50,000 a year pays $350 a month for individual coverage in an HMO. If such an individual wants to buy the plan that allows her to choose any doctor, she may pay $450 a month. In the same city, a self-employed person with a spouse and two or three children may pay upwards of $600 a month for insurance. Is it any wonder many people are reeling under the financial burden of health insurance, while being increasingly dissatisfied with the care paid for by "affordable" insurance?

Medical savings accounts (MSAs) are a relatively new instrument of paying for health care and they offer the freedom and flexibility that patients need. By the end of the year 2000, Congress was to have legislated clear guidelines as to who is eligible and what amount of the plan is tax deductible. Basically, the concept is health insurance with a high deductible. Depending on the state where you live, it is about $2,000 for an individual, and $4,000 for a family. Again depending on where you live, the premiums are around $175 for an individual and $225 for a family.

This is coupled with a tax-deductible savings account at a financial institution offering MSA accounts. A percentage of the insurance premium is paid into the account each month or quarter. The cost of the premium and the deposit to the savings account should about equal the cost of the better HMO plans. However, you are free to go to any physician you want. The account can be used to pay the first medical costs that are not met by the high deductible or it can be saved for greater expenses. At the end of each year, whatever monies have not been spent are rolled over into the next year. The money in the account is yours or your family's to use for health expenses, from deductibles to eyeglasses to root canals. To find the name of an agent who sells MSAs in your state, contact the National Association of Alternative Brokers at 1-800-627-0552.

I am aware of the fact that millions of low-income Americans have neither the insurance nor the financial means to obtain proper diagnosis and treatment. In the past, before medicine became so expensive, before its domination by managed care, physicians had more time to devote to caring for the poor or underinsured. They spent less time on the "business" of medicine.

Nevertheless, there are physicians who still make the effort to care for the underinsured or financially disadvantaged. It is still possible in our health-care system for low-income Americans to obtain good quality care, usually in such arenas as public or Veterans Hospitals staffed by a medical school. This is a far from perfect solution to the inequalities of the human condition. It is also a testimony to the need for change in the American health-care system.

Getting the Most from Your Health-Insurance Plan

Money does not always buy quality, but it helps. The least expensive doctors in your plan are not necessarily the best or the worst. However, if you consult with an experienced pain specialist who charges enough money to be able to focus on your problems for sixty minutes, as opposed to one who sees two or three patients in that time, you are likely to receive better care.

If you have a long-standing pain problem that has not been adequately treated by various other physicians within your network or by physicians whom you consider affordable or geographically convenient, it may be time to look elsewhere and spend more money out of pocket. This also applies to patients covered by insurance companies rather than managed-care plans. Many insurance companies balk at paying for high-quality care to diagnose and treat many painful conditions, because many of these conditions are test-negative and there are no objective tests to prove the severity of a patient's pain.

In this era of increased emphasis on cutting health-care costs, insurance carriers can view pain management as an elective luxury treatment, similar to cosmetic surgery or long-term psychotherapy. Therefore, some insurance companies frequently reimburse insufficiently or refuse to pay for pain-management services for the same reasons they pay little or nothing for psychiatric services, another subjective gray area in medicine.

Some insurers limit the amount of certain pain-relieving drugs patients may obtain on their plan in a given period of time. Many insurance companies do not reimburse much for costly, invasive pain-management procedures. For example, some policies will only cover two or three nerve blocks in one year, even though a patient may need six blocks to obtain a full evaluation of a painful condition, and another procedure involving six radiofrequency lesions to obtain long-term pain relief. Current insurance policies often result in insufficient pain control, forcing certain patients to either suffer or spend their own funds to obtain adequate pain relief.

Your doctor may help you appeal your insurance company's decisions, but ultimately you have a contract with your insurance company and must decide how you want to deal with the limitations of your coverage. You may have to pay a small or large portion of your doctor's fee out of your pocket in order to obtain the pain relief you desire.

Do not join with your insurer or health-care network in being penny wise and pound foolish in terms of your health. Remember, an insurance company makes money by holding on to your premiums for as long as possible, gaining interest on them, and paying as little and as slowly as possible for your health care. Their primary goal must be to earn as much money as possible, not to improve your health. They are more accountable to their stockholders than to you, the patient.

Patients in chronic pain clearly represent a complicated problem that may not be adequately addressed by the volume-driven system of today. Anyone in pain for more than six months despite so-called adequate care by a physician should look for, and be prepared to pay for, high-quality consultants for second opinions. If you are contemplating going on disability because of poorly controlled pain, consult other specialists first, while you still can. Remember, once you become disabled, you may remain in that state—while your pain, depression, anxiety, frustration, anger, economic situation, and even your marriage and other relationships get gradually and inexorably worse.

FINDING THE BEST DOCTOR

Any physician engaged in pain management should be trained rigorously in the diagnosis and medical and surgical treatment of various painful conditions within such specialties as neurology, neurosurgery, oncology, rheumatology, and orthopedics to name a few. This includes evaluating patients by eliciting a thorough history of their complaints. This is an art in itself, and when supplemented by a focused physical examination and diagnostic tests is most likely to provide the correct diagnosis regarding the cause of pain. The diagnosis guides the treatment and predicts the short- and long-term outcome for the patient. Misdiagnosis could result in prolonged mismanagement of pain, the cause of which could be medically or effectively treated or eliminated.

Pain should be treated during the diagnostic evaluation and subsequent treatment. It should be definitely be controlled on a chronic basis if no diagnosis is found, or no medical or surgical treatment directed at its purported cause relieves it.

Anesthesiologists, neurologists, rheumatologists, physiatrists, psychiatrists, some orthopedists, and neurosurgeons are all involved in pain management, in a fragmented alliance held together by a common interest in relieving pain. Anesthesiologists, neurosurgeons, and recently some physiatrists use more surgical procedures than those physicians from the medical and psychiatric specialties. Procedure-oriented physicians may rely more on interventional procedures than their pill-prescribing medical colleagues. Both approaches to a complicated pain problem may be useful, depending on the problem and patient.

There are 925,000 licensed physicians in the United States, of which only an estimated four thousand have any training in controlling intractable pain. Some of these four thousand physicians may agree to prescribe opiates on a chronic basis, while others may just perform pain-relieving procedures such as blocks or neurosurgery. Here are some clues to the kind of pain treatment you are likely to find.

- Anesthesiologists are the most likely to use nerve blocks, epidurals, and, depending on the physician, other pain-relieving procedures including spinal-cord stimulation, implanted pumps, and cryoanalgesia or radiofrequency-lesioning techniques for pain control.

- Neurosurgeons involved in pain control are likely to use radiofrequency procedures on certain nerves involving the spine as well as procedures to selectively destroy pain pathways in the brain and spinal cord. They may also implant spinal-cord and brain stimulators and drug pumps.

- Some orthopedists interested in spinal problems may use epidurals and some are beginning to evaluate and treat low-back pain by performing discography and other procedures to relieve discogenic pain. Some perform vertebroplasty.

- Radiologists do not evaluate pain problems but may be asked to perform a specific procedure by another physician treating a pain patient. Some radiologists may perform facet blocks, nerve-root blocks, epidurals, discograms, celiac plexus blocks (for pancreatic and abdominal pain), and verte-broplasty, all procedures performed with the help of X-ray machines to visualize the placement of needles within the body.

- Most neurologists, physiatrists, rheumatologists, and psychiatrists will treat pain with medication. (Unfortunately, at present, very few neurologists treat patients with interventional pain-relieving procedures.)

- Physiatrists also will use physical therapy, including trigger-point injections. A small but growing number of physiatrists utilize interventional pain-management procedures including nerve blocks, facet blocks, discograms, and some cryoanalgesia and radiofrequency-lesioning procedures.

- Psychiatrists and psychologists, naturally, use psychotherapy and behavioral techniques.

- Neurologists, neurosurgeons, and some orthopedists specializing in spinal disorders may be the most likely to diagnose and treat spinal-pain problems. The latter two specialists perform surgery, and some of them may be more likely to advise surgery than a more conservative neurologist. At times either approach—surgery or conservative care—is appropriate. Sometimes one is better. Thus, you need to see various doctors and get various opinions.

- Neurologists and neurosurgeons are most likely to diagnose neuropathic pain, with the exception of some unusual cases of CRPS, in which case certain pain specialists (usually a neurologist, anesthesiologist, or neurosurgeon with special expertise in this painful disorder) may provide better guidance.

- Musculoskeletal pain, including sports injuries, arthritis, fibromyalgia, and osteoporosis, may be best diagnosed and treated by rheumatologists, physiatrists, and orthopedists. Sports injuries should be evaluated and treated by specialists in sports medicine.

- Endocrinologists specializing in bone disorders also treat osteoporosis.

- Cancer- and AIDS-related pain is best diagnosed and treated by oncologists, neurologists, and other pain-management specialists with training in cancer and AIDS.

Pain can make you crazy, and so can our health-care system. Who wants to spend thirty dollars on parking and three hundred dollars on pills, wait hours in a doctor's office, and then undergo an operation only to find out the treatment doesn't work? This is why you must take responsibility for actively choosing your doctors. Following the line of least resistance, particularly when it is advocated by managed-care organizations, will not necessarily get you the treatment you need.

Once you've done the research and found some doctors you believe might be able to help you, talk to them before you decide. Interview the doctor on the phone or in person. If you expect to have a lengthy conversation with the physician on the telephone, be prepared to pay for the doctor's time. I ask patients to fill out a detailed questionnaire (by mail or on my Web site) and send me their X rays and other records to help me decide if I feel I can help them. Ask physicians the questions below. Hopefully the information in this book will help you evaluate their answers.

- How many patients with my physical complaint have you treated?

- Were they treated with noninvasive, conservative methods like medication, physical therapy, TENS, and acupuncture? If that failed, what was the next step?

- How long should I undergo conservative treatment before trying invasive pain treatments or surgery?

- How do you decide whether to treat me with invasive techniques like nerve blocks, epidurals, facet blocks, discography, radiofrequency lesioning, cryoanalgesia, procedures designed to lessen disk-related pain, vertebroplasty, spinal-cord or peripheral-nerve stimulation, implantable pumps, and invasive neurosurgical methods of pain control?

- In what order do you try them—in other words, if one fails, how would you go up the rungs of the ladder to the next?

- What are the short- and long-term risks of someone like me taking medication or undergoing any invasive procedure?

Here is another set of questions to ask if you are talking with a doctor about surgery:

- What conditions do you feel are best treated surgically, and how do you diagnose these conditions?

- If I am a candidate for surgery, what surgical treatments do you suggest for my condition?

- If you are not a spine surgeon, what surgeons do you recommend?

- Do I really need a fusion or can I get by quite well with a simpler operation like a discectomy or foramenotomy?

Once your doctor has prescribed a particular treatment, ask about alternatives. If he or she resists answering your questions, change doctors! You do have choices, but you may have to step outside your system to get them. Find out what the long-term results of this physician's treatment are and how they compare with results published by other doctors using the same methods in similar patients. Getting better for only a few hours, days, weeks, or even months from an invasive treatment designed to provide years of relief is not enough. Ask:

- Were most patients with conditions like mine significantly relieved or cured of their pain for years? If not, what became of them?

- What percentage of similar patients were able to decrease their medication usage and increase their activity by 50 percent for years following treatment? What became of the other patients?

Ask your doctor for a list of references and ask for names of some patients for whom his or her treatments did work and also some for whom they did not work. I provide these to my patients. If a doctor is offended by this idea, he or she may not be the right doctor for you. Ask these patients the following:

- Did the treatment really help?

- Was it worth the cost and inconvenience?

- How did the outcome change your life?

- What was the actual procedure like?

- What was the facility like where the procedure was performed?

By speaking to patients whose treatment failed, you will be able to tell how the physician manages patients who are treatment failures. Did the physician abandon them or direct them to another source of help?

Finally, what is the doctor's staff like? A great doctor with a somewhat disorganized office is something you can live with, even if the physician should not. However, it helps to know about this in advance.

In the Doctor's Office

At the doctor's office, a staff member will provide you with a form to fill out describing your pain. Not only should these forms help you list your insurers, medical history, and your other physicians, they should help you articulate your condition.

You should be asked to state the site of your pain and you should be offered adjectives to describe it: aching, throbbing, burning, shooting, stabbing, pulling, cramping, dull, sharp, intermittent, constant, fluctuating in severity. State the positions or activities that make it worse and better, how it has changed over time, and how it affects your sleep.

Patients in pain, especially the depressed and the elderly, cannot always present their cases in a meaningful way that helps the doctor zero in on their problem. Carefully filling out the intake form is a help to doctor and patient. If you need help doing so, ask a friend or relative for help. Certainly the doctor's staff should be of help as well.

Sometimes chronic-pain patients are suspected of faking or exaggerating their problem in order to obtain monetary, psychological, or social support or to gain access to narcotics. Very few chronic-pain patients are guilty of any or all of these abuses. However, some pain-management physicians may unwittingly contribute to such abuses if they don't refer patients who clearly exaggerate their symptoms to psychiatrists. A few physicians may try one expensive pain therapy after another for patients who are motivated to remain in the "sick" role.

Most chronic-pain patients, especially those still active in work and family and social life, have no hidden agenda. They simply hurt and want to get better. They will go to great lengths to lessen their pain so as to lead a fuller life. The majority of pain specialists try very hard to use their expertise, medication and procedures, and compassion to help their patients improve.

Being a Partner in Your Health Care

A physician has the responsibility to correctly diagnose a patient and treat him or her as effectively as possible, given the patient's medical and psychological condition. However, in working with the usual pain patient that I see, who has already been to several other colleagues, the "we try harder" motto comes to mind. These patients are not spending their good time and money to have me tell them that their problem, which I may not always immediately understand, is "all in their head," or that they should try a third course of physical therapy despite the fact that the other two didn't work, or that they "will have to live with it."

Therefore, in my specialty, compassion, patience, dogged determination to resolve a problem, and intelligence and creativity in seeking solutions are absolutely essential to success—and to my own professional and personal satisfaction. I am not the only physician who thinks this way. Find your own. But find one who takes you seriously.

In working with your doctor to maximize your treatment, think of what you can do instead of what you cannot. What can you do around the house, even with some degree of discomfort? What act of kindness have you undertaken for anyone in your family, circle of friends, or community? Patients in pain, or with any other debilitating illness, may drift into desperation and depression.

It is critical to stay connected to life, to your family and friends, to your local church, temple, mosque, or community organizations, and possibly to see a psychotherapist. I knew a wonderful man who was dying of emphysema. In his last weeks as he lay in bed, he would call the florist to send his wife flowers. If he couldn't dial the phone, he would get someone else to do it. He was connected to his life outside the hospital until the very end.

Chronic-pain sufferers aren't dying, but some will have good and bad days for the rest of their lives. For these patients, no matter what is done to minimize the level of pain when it flares, there will still be some days where pain is moderate as opposed to mild or nonexistent.

Part of being a patient is being realistic about what medicine can and can't do for you and what you can and cannot do to help yourself. Physicians have to be equally realistic. Sometimes even patients I help significantly—but perhaps not enough—leave me to shop for other doctors. I am not offended. In fact, I am always curious about learning from my mistakes. If another doctor could help a patient better than I, then I wanted to know about the treatment. However, because I have a great deal of experience, I am correct most of the time. If I feel a patient has reached maximum improvement, I am generally correct. Both the patient and I must accept the limitations of present-day medicine and life in general. Medicine and surgery are not cures for the aging process, for example.

The elderly, overweight, disabled or unemployed, depressed or anxious, habitual users of high dosages of pain medications, and those who have undergone many surgical procedures respond less well to treatment for long-standing pain than others. They can be helped, but the path to relief is more complicated. They can be made more comfortable, but they are unlikely to be completely cured.

My patient Albert injured his back in a traffic accident, yet he still delivers industrial foam each day. I respect him for working with his pain—for not ceding to the disabling demands of his pain, for fighting to find something, someone to make him better. Yet when he comes to my office he is in a desperate emotional state and breaks down in tears because he can't pick up his daughter and he is furious that I cannot completely cure him. I performed a diagnostic nerve block that gave him relief for longer than I expected, and when it wore off he called my office on a weekend and was angry that I wasn't personally available. Later, my office tried to return his call five times, but he was never in. Then he was furious that we hadn't called him. He said he was sick and tired of being in pain. Chronically sick patients may become childlike.

Pain flavors every aspect of his life from the time he gets up to the time when he goes to bed. However, I think there are some reasonable boundaries patients need to observe if they are going to get the most from a doctor and his or her medical staff. You can complain about drugs that don't work and cause side effects and about drugs that do work but cause side effects. You are supposed to tell me honestly about the outcome of your procedures and whether you have tremendous postoperative pain. But patients are not entitled to be abusive to my staff or me. They rarely are.

However, sometimes we do see people who are so angry, depressed, and desperate about being in chronic pain that they need psychiatric help in dealing with their pain and its effects on their life. My problem is when such patients refuse such therapy and continue to be abusive or unable to participate in their own care to an optimal degree. There is nothing that I, or anyone else, can do for someone who refuses treatment, or follows suggestions for treatment halfheartedly. I usually recommend that such patients find another physician to work with on a long-standing basis.

Above all, the important thing to know is that you do have a choice in medical care. The only question is whether you will undertake the responsibilities of claiming that choice and getting the best possible care.

If you are reading this book, I am sure you will make that choice.

KEY POINTS
About Finding the Best Care

- If you have doubts about a doctor's ability to treat your pain effectively, go to another doctor—even if you have to pay for it out of pocket.

- Be as accurate as you can in describing your pain and the treatment you have tried so far.

- Expect your doctor to take you seriously and believe that you are in pain.

- If your health-insurance company refuses to pay for particular tests or treatment that you need, make an appeal in writing or through a specialized attorney, if needed.

- Consider changing your medical coverage to an insurer who gives you a choice of any medical care you want, even if it costs more.

AFTERWORD

A little rebellion now and then is a good thing.
—THOMAS JEFFERSON

I've given you a lot of information to absorb in these pages, but if you've been paying attention, you know that I feel passionately that people in pain have a right to the best treatment they can find, and our current health-care system is making that just about impossible.

We need to educate everyone—the medical profession, insurance companies, the public, and legislators—about types of pain, personal and cultural responses to pain, test-negative and referred pain, and the prevention of chronic pain syndrome, with all its attendant psychological, social, and economic baggage. Some drastic changes are needed before we can have the kind of health care that we need—for everyone—patients as well as doctors.

In 1989, Dr. John Bonica, a founding father of the whole field of pain medicine, said, "No medical school has a pain curriculum." Given the widespread level of ignorance and misinformation on pain, a primary reason for patients to visit doctors, we should conclude that patients do not have intractable pain, but they may have intractable doctors.

Medical students learn about the neurological structures that process pain and the mechanisms by which these structures receive, transmit, and modulate pain impulses. However, they get little exposure to methods of controlling pain. While they learn about the pharmacology of various drugs useful in pain control, that pharmacology class does not teach them how to use drugs in a clinical setting with real people.

Once out of school, fledgling physicians learn how to practice medicine from the interns and residents with whom they train and from the attending physicians teaching them clinical medicine and surgery. Unfortunately, too often young physicians learn early in their careers that treatment of pain is subordinate to surgical or medical treatment of disease.

The cycle can only be broken through initiatives in which pain specialists in medical schools teach students about pain control. For the senior physicians in hospitals and training programs, attendance at pain-management courses should be a mandatory prerequisite to being allowed to practice in a given hospital. Hospital admitting privileges should be given only to those doctors who pass a test on the basic principles of pain control. Such a program would cajole physicians into taking pain more seriously and diagnosing and treating it more effectively, including through the use of narcotics. Physicians should also learn when to send patients to pain specialists for treatment, to help control severe pain. Programs already exist in some states and hospitals to educate physicians in areas such as infection control and the recognition of domestic, child, and elder abuse.

Pain must also be considered a vital sign in all hospital and doctor's offices, the same as temperature, pulse, and blood pressure. There is a trend in this direction, and I hope it continues. Just as you don't have to and should not live with high blood pressure, you should not have to live in severe or even moderate chronic pain. I favor the creation of a formally recognized specialty devoted to pain management, in which physicians in a residency study all the aspects of diagnosing and treating the gamut of painful disorders. This would obviate the need for patients to choose an appropriate specialist to obtain pain relief. Unfortunately at present, this decision is often made somewhat arbitrarily with predictable consequences.

We need basic research into the anatomical, biochemical, and molecular basis of poorly understood pain syndromes, such as fibromyalgia, CPRS, and chronic back pain, to name a few, some of which are test-negative using today's conventional diagnostic armamentarium. Improved understanding of these disorders would go a long way to improve compassionate acceptance and treatment of patients suffering from them by the skeptics in the medical community, as well as by the insurance companies.

Physical pain is a symptom of a disease process and, in some cases, may be a complicated disease itself. Usually it is not simply a form of psychological disturbance. Yet because the basis for so many painful disorders is unknown, the treatments for these disorders are poorly defined. We must pursue research on the mechanisms underlying chronic pain. New drugs to control difficult-to-treat neuropathic pain, narcotics with fewer side effects, and other, cleaner drugs to help us modulate pain must be developed. There is a considerable amount of exciting research in this area, and on behalf of my patients, I hope it will be facilitated with appropriate public and private support.

As you know, I and most doctors—and probably most patients—are enraged about the way American health care has been downgraded. Is anybody in the world getting better treatment? We don't know. We do know patients are becoming statistics and not getting the quality of care they need, and doctors are dropping out because they cannot practice real medicine anymore.

Rather than let the insurance companies decide what treatments they will pay for, we might look at the entire issue another way. Let's pay for treatment based on outcomes. Instead of giving doctors and hospitals an incentive to provide unnecessary surgery because it pays more than a less invasive procedure, why not reimburse both physicians and surgeons based on outcome—prorated to the complexity of the patient's problems? The same policy should be directed at pain management and even diagnostic tests. Physicians' fees and hospital reimbursement for treatment that achieves the best long-term results at the least long-term cost should be higher than for comparatively less effective therapy. Recently the Central Florida Health Care Coalition proposed reimbursing physicians on the basis of treatment outcome for various conditions including low-back pain, as well as on evidence that the physicians were keeping abreast of the latest developments in their field. Clearly, the means by which the difficulty of the condition is prorated and outcome is measured are important methodological issues to tackle in such a scheme. However, this proposal represents a positive trend in health-care reimbursement.

Outcome can be measured by studying function and quality of life, using specialty- or disease-specific standardized tests and taking into account the type, frequency, and cost of interaction with the health-care system following a given treatment. In the case of spinal surgery, the extent and type of removal of a disk or stenosis could be evaluated by radiologists and correlated with postoperative function by a neurologist, for example—someone other than the surgeon.

The same sort of follow-up could be applied to various types of pain treatment, and also should be evaluated by an independent physician capable of judging the success of treatment. The utility and quality of diagnostic tests could be substantiated in a similar manner. For example, I estimate that in most spine-related pain disorders, 90 percent of the electrical diagnostic tests are unnecessary. The diagnosis usually can be based on a good history and physical examination and an excellent radiological evaluation of the spinal anatomy. Similarly, poor-quality, cheap MRIs, which do not demonstrate anatomy accurately enough for a doctor to make a correct surgical decision, may be identified as a "false economy" by such a system, because the procedure often has to be performed again, using a better MRI.

We advance in medicine by learning from our successes and our failures. Outcome analysis is the only real way of keeping us "honest," allowing us to learn what really does and doesn't work to treat a given problem. The source of pain is often exceedingly difficult to diagnose and treat. Despite our best efforts, much pain is not controlled successfully. We need all the feedback we can get to help our patients maintain a high-quality, satisfying life and stay far away from that slippery one-way tunnel down to the inferno of chronic disability.

There are many stories of people in pain in this book. For their sake, and for the millions like them, I hope we can make some real progress into a new understanding of why it is so important to treat pain on a higher level than currently exists.

Although medical excellence isn't necessary to treat the common cold, it is necessary to treat most of the problems described in this book. I insist on it. I feel my profession should, too—through collective action, if necessary. And I have tried to provide suggestions—medical, social, and financial—to allow you and your family to obtain excellent care.

GLOSSARY

Acupuncture: a traditional Chinese therapeutic process in which specific points of the body are stimulated with needles to foster healing or pain relief.

Addiction: compulsive use of a drug for psychological purposes, such as mood alteration. This is distinct from scheduled use of a given dose of a drug for medical purposes, such as pain relief. (Also see *pseudoaddiction.*)

Analgesia: relief of pain.

Anesthesia: loss of sensation. Also a treatment that causes controlled analgesia, amnesia or recollection of events, and muscular relaxation.

Anesthesiologist: a physician who specializes in using medications that provide pain relief, relaxation, and lack of awareness during painful procedures. Anesthesiologists also monitor and maintain a patient's vital functions during this time. They also manage pain for a few days following procedures. Some may also manage chronic painful conditions.

Annulus: The leathery covering of a disk surrounding the nucleus, or rubbery core.

Antidepressant: a medication used to treat depression. Some antidepressants may also be used to treat pain.

Arachnoid: the spiderweblike covering of the brain, spinal cord, cauda equina, and nerve roots.

Arachnoiditis: inflammation and scarring of the arachnoid, at times causing pain, numbness, and weakness in the legs and bowel, bladder, and sexual dysfunction. Arachnoiditis may be caused by spinal surgery, usually without serious consequences, or by old myelograms, with potentially serious results.

Autonomic nervous system: the part of the nervous system that functions in an automatic, unconscious fashion, regulating bodily functions such as heart rate, blood pressure, sweating, and digestion, for example.

Avulsion: forceful separation of connected parts, i.e., a root is ripped free of the spinal cord.

Axon: the part of a nerve cell that delivers impulses from that cell to other cells.

Block: an injection of a chemical that blocks or stops the transmission of nerve impulses, resulting in possible pain relief, numbness, weakness, and other phenomena. These may be performed for diagnostic (to determine what is the cause of pain) or therapeutic (to alleviate pain) purposes.

CAT (computerized axial tomography) scan: a diagnostic radiological technique combining a computer and X rays passed through the body at various angles. It provides detailed three-dimensional information about the structure of the body.

Cauda equina: Latin for *horse's tail*. This is a group of nerve roots exiting the end of the spinal cord in the upper lumbar spine. These roots control the muscle power and sensation of the lower extremities as well as bowel, bladder, and sexual function.

Cell body: the main part of a nerve cell.

Central nervous system: the brain and spinal cord, which receive and process sensory information from the rest of the body and respond by initiating muscle movement or some other response.

Cervical: pertaining to the neck.

Complex regional pain syndrome (CRPS): a type of chronic neuropathic pain, also previously known as reflex sympathetic dystrophy (RSD). It is characterized by burning pain; changes in skin color, temperature, and texture; and deterioration of the vitality of the musculoskeletal system in the affected area.

Compression fracture: collapse of a bone (often a vertebral body) caused by trauma or by weakening from osteoporosis or cancer.

Corticosteroids: active hormones produced by the adrenal glands, producing biological effects on various bodily systems. Man-made analogues to these hormones possess potent anti-inflammatory and pain-relieving properties and cause considerable side effects.

Cranial: pertaining to the head. Cranial nerves are those peripheral nerves which have their origins in the brain. Most of them function primarily on structures in the head.

Dependence: the body's adaptation to the presence of a drug, such as narcotics, alcohol, caffeine, and nicotine. When a person is dependent on a chemical, the lack of it causes withdrawal symptoms.

Dendrite: part(s) of a nerve cell that receive incoming impulses from other nerve cells.

Disk: flattened circular structure something like a checker piece with a soft core. They lie between the vertebral bodies of the spine.

Discectomy: a surgical procedure to remove disk material, usually following disk herniation.

Discogenic: originating in the disk.

Discogram: procedure to determine which disks cause pain. Radiological dye is injected into a disk and indicates the structural condition of the interior of the disk and its covering.

Dorsal: pertaining to the back of the body, i.e., a dorsal root enters the back of the spinal cord.

Dorsal Root Entry Zone (DREZ): the part of the spinal cord into which pain impulses from peripheral nerves enter the central nervous system. Damage to this zone can cause pain, as in postherpetic neuralgia, and neurosurgically induced lesions here can relieve it, as in a DREZ procedure.

Dura: tough external covering of the brain, spinal cord, cauda equina, and nerve roots. Under the dura are the arachnoid, spinal fluid, and nervous system structures.

Dye: pertaining to radiological dye, also known as contrast. This injected liquid is used to enhance the information gained from various radiological tests, including myelograms and some CAT scans. A special form of contrast is used to enhance MRI images.

Dysfunction: improper or abnormal function.

Electromyogram (EMG): an electrical diagnostic test. This is usually combined with a nerve conduction velocity (NCV) examination. Together they are used to evaluate disorders of the spinal nerve roots, peripheral nerves, and muscles.

Endorphins: hormones or chemical substances manufactured by the body that relieve pain and produce euphoria. They are opioids, acting like drugs derived from opium (narcotics).

Epidural: pertaining to the area within the spinal canal outside the dura. It contains fat and veins.

Euphoria: a feeling of happiness and well-being.

Facet: a joint supporting the spine. Facets are located on either side of the spine and connect each vertebra to those above and below.

Fascia: a layer of connective tissue surrounding the muscles of the body.

Fibromyalgia: a diffuse, painful condition characterized by tender areas within muscles. It is not to be confused with myofascial pain, which is less diffuse and is associated with smaller focal areas of muscle tenderness.

Flexion-extension X rays: X rays used to evaluate the degree of slippage of one vertebra over another. These X rays are taken from the side with the patient bending forward (flexes) and backward (extends) in order to determine the stability of the spine during this kind of movement.

Foramen (plural: foramina): holes on either side of the spine through which the spinal roots exit the spinal canal.

Fusion: an operation in which one or more vertebrae of the spine are fused together with another piece of bone or metal hardware.

Ganglion (plural: ganglia): a mass of cell bodies of sensory or autonomic nerves. Each spinal root and certain cranial nerves have a ganglion. There are various autonomic ganglia near the spine and in other parts of the body.

Gastrointestinal: pertaining to the digestive tract.

Herniate: the projection of tissue through a defect in surrounding tissue. In a disk herniation, the rubbery core of the disk pushes through the annulus. Sometimes, but not always, this material presses on a nerve and causes pain.

Horse's tail: see *Cauda equina*.

Inflammation: reaction by the body involving local swelling, increased temperature, pain, and red coloration of the affected tissues. It is a response to damage, including infection.

Interventional: pertaining to invasive procedures, in which the body is penetrated with a needle or probe or opened surgically.

Intraspinal: inside the spinal canal. In this book, this term refers to drug delivery either into the epidural space or spinal fluid.

Intravenous: pertaining to delivery of a substance into a vein.

Invasive: pertaining to procedures involving penetration of or entry into the body.

Lamina: one of the two sides of the arch arising from the vertebral body. The arch makes up the back of the spinal canal.

Laminectomy: removal of one arch of a vertebra.

Laminotomy: removal of part of one arch of a vertebra.

Lesioning: partial or complete destruction of nerve tissue. In this book, lesions are made for the purpose of ending or moderating the pain messages sent by those nerves to the brain.

Ligamentum flavum: Latin for "yellow ligament." These are the ligaments inside the spinal canal, which stabilize the spine. They bulge and become hard with calcium deposits with age, causing narrowing of the spinal canal and exerting pressure on the nerve roots.

Local anesthetic: a chemical that is placed in contact with nervous tissue and reduces the ability of nerves to transmit impulses, including those carrying pain messages.

Lumbar: having to do with the lower spine between the lowest rib and the pelvis.

Medical: as pertains to therapy, nonsurgical treatment, usually involving medication.

Molecule: the basic unit of any chemical made up of more than one element.

Morphine: a narcotic analgesic or painkiller derived from the opium poppy.

Motor: pertaining to muscle contraction and movement.

MRI (magnetic resonance imaging): a diagnostic technique that provides three-dimensional images of the structure of the body through exposure to a magnetic field, without the use of radiation.

Musculoskeletal: pertaining to ligaments, tendons, muscle, or bone. Musculoskeletal pain arises from these structures and in such disorders as arthritis, fibromyalgia, myofascial pain, most back and neck pain, some headaches, temporomandibular-joint pain, and some cancer pain.

Myelogram: a diagnostic test in which radiological dye is injected into the spinal fluid; X rays and usually CAT scans are taken to evaluate sources of pressure on the spinal cord and nerve roots (such as disk herniations, stenosis, spinal slippage).

Myofascial pain: pain related to focal areas of muscle contraction.

Narcotics: a class of drug that binds to specific receptors within the body that are also bound to by endorphins, our naturally occurring narcoticlike chemicals. Narcotics are used to relieve moderate to severe pain.

Neuralgia: pain traveling along the course of a nerve or nerves that is caused by dysfunction or damage to the nerve(s) involved in the pain.

Neurologist: a physician specializing in the diagnosis and medical treatment of diseases and disorders of the nervous system. A few subspecialize in the drug-related treatment of pain.

Neuroma: a focal mass of scar tissue arising from a damaged nerve.

Neuron: a nerve cell. A neuron is composed of a cell body, dendrites, and an axon.

Neuropathic: pertaining to pain or unpleasant sensation caused by nervous-system dysfunction or injury.

Neuropathy: disease of the peripheral nerves, often causing sensory loss, pain, or weakness. Neuropathy may involve one or more nerves.

Neurosurgeon: a physician specializing in the surgical treatment of nervous-system diseases and disorders. A few subspecialize in the treatment of pain through interventional procedures.

Neurotransmitter: a chemical that carries messages between neurons or nerve cells.

NSAIDs (nonsteroidal anti-inflammatory drugs): a type of painkilling drugs that reduce inflammation. They block the production of prostaglandins, chemicals that cause inflammation and initiate pain. Aspirin is the most common NSAID. Tylenol (acetaminophen) is not an NSAID.

Nucleus: the rubbery central portion of a disk.

Opiate: a drug derived from opium.

Opioid: a drug that acts like an opiate.

Orthopedist: a physician specializing in the surgical treatment of conditions of the bones, joints, muscles, tendons, and ligaments.

Pain: an unpleasant sensory or emotional experience, not necessarily associated with damage to the body.

PCA (patient-controlled analgesia): a method of pain relief in which patients are allowed to self-administer pain medication, usually by controlling the schedule by which they receive their medication. This method usually involves a device attached to an intravenous infusion but may be used with subcutaneous or intraspinal drug delivery.

Peripheral nervous system: all the nerves carrying sensory and motor impulses to and from the central nervous system and the rest of the body.

Pharmacological: pertaining to drugs or chemicals with medically important biological effects.

Pharmacology: a scientific diskipline that deals with the design and function of chemicals that exert biological effects and that can be exploited medically.

Physiatrist: a physician specializing in rehabilitation and the use of physical medicine. Some physiatrists subspecialize in treating chronic pain.

Physical medicine: nonpharmacological, noninvasive, manual or mechanical methods to promote pain relief and increase function. These include physical therapy, braces, splints, externally applied heat or cold, ultrasound, external electrical stimulation, and massage, for example.

Physical therapist: a specially trained and licensed medical professional who performs physical therapy. A physical therapist is not a physician and is supposed to provide physical-therapeutic treatment only under prescription of a physician.

Postherpetic neuralgia: chronic pain at the site of an attack of shingles.

Prolapse: in this book, this pertains to bulging of the nucleus or center of a disk and an overlying area in the covering of the disk or annulus. This condition is less severe than a herniation.

Pseudoaddiction: drug-seeking (usually narcotic-seeking) behavior by a patient suffering from inadequately treated pain. The narcotics are sought for pain relief, not for psychological purposes, which would represent true addiction.

Psychiatrist: a physician who specializes in the diagnosis and treatment of disorders of thought, emotion, and behavior. Treatment may include psychotherapy, medication, and rarely surgery on the brain. Some psychiatrists have special expertise in working with chronic-pain patients.

Psychologist: a licensed mental-health professional who practices psychotherapy. Psychologists do not have a medical degree and cannot prescribe medication.

Psychotherapist: an individual who performs psychotherapy. Certain psychiatrists, clinical psychologists, certain social workers, and others may be considered psychotherapists.

Psychotherapy: nonpharmacological, nonsurgical, usually verbally based treatment for disorders of thought, emotion, or behavior.

Radicular pain: pain that radiates from a painful focus. Pain caused by root irritation or dysfunction also is referred to as radicular. (*Radicle* is the Latin origin of *root*.)

Radiofrequency: a type of energy which can be harnessed to produce heat. Using appropriate equipment, it can be used to achieve exquisitely localized, partial or complete destruction of tissue, including nerves.

Radiological: pertaining to radiology, the medical specialty that obtains and interprets images of the internal structure of the body.

Radiologist: a physician who is trained in obtaining and interpreting images of the internal structure of the body with specialized diagnostic equipment, such as X rays, magnetic resonance imaging, and sound waves (ultrasound).

Receptor: a three-dimensional structure composed of large molecules, often on the surface of a cell, to which other specific three-dimensional molecules (drugs, neurotransmitters, and hormones) can bind in a "lock and key" interaction. This interaction may produce a biological effect, such as an increase or decrease in the impulses generated by a nerve cell containing the receptor.

Referred pain: pain transmitted to an area distant from its cause.

Reflex sympathetic dystrophy (RSD): See *complex regional pain syndrome.*

Rheumatologist: a physician who diagnoses and treats arthritis and other conditions involving the joints, muscles, or connective tissues.

Root: the portion of a nerve running between the spinal cord and foramen. Once the root exits the foramen, it is simply called a nerve. Roots are also referred to as spinal roots or nerve roots in this book.

Side effect: an unwanted effect of a drug.

Spinal canal: the space within the spine through which course the spinal cord, roots, and their coverings. It is composed of the arch of the vertebra behind and the rear of the body in the front.

Spinal cord: the part of the central nervous system extending from the brain down to the upper lumbar spine. It serves to bring messages about the body (sensation) from the roots up to the brain and bring messages from the brain down to the roots, from which these messages travel out to the peripheral nerves and affect the body.

Spinal fluid: a clear, colorless, waterlike fluid bathing the spinal cord and brain.

Spine: the column of bones, disks, and ligaments running from the base of the skull to the pelvis and enclosing the spinal cord, cauda equina, and nerve roots.

Stenosis: narrowing of a passage in the body. In this book, stenosis pertains to narrowing of the spinal canal or foramina due to arthritic overgrowth, disk bulges or herniation, bulging ligaments, or spinal slippage.

Subcutaneous: under the skin.

Sympathetic: pertaining to a part of the autonomic nervous system. Historically, the sympathetic nerves have been implicated in the pain and dysfunction of what was called reflex sympathetic dystrophy and is now called complex regional pain syndrome.

Temporomandibular: pertaining to the joints of the jaw, connecting the jaw (mandible) to the temporal bone of the skull. Temporomandibular-joint pain affects the local area of the joint and may radiate out into the nearby face and head and down into the neck.

TENS (transcutaneous electrical nerve stimulation): a form of pain-relieving therapy in which mild electrical stimulation from a portable device is delivered to the skin through small electrodes glued to the skin.

Test-negative pain: pain that has no cause that can be detected by plain X rays, CAT scans, MRIs, electrical tests, or laboratory-based diagnostic tools. This type of pain may be investigated with diagnostic nerve blocks and discograms.

Tic douleureux: see *trigeminal neuralgia.*

Thoracic: pertaining to the chest area, or that part of the spine to which the ribs are attached.

Tolerance: the body's adaptation to a drug so that the drug has fewer beneficial effects and side effects.

Trigger point: a small knotted bundle of fibers within a muscle that is the cause of myofascial muscle pain.

Trigeminal neuralgia: a form of neuropathic pain in which pain impulses arise from the trigeminal or fifth cranial nerve, its ganglion, or its connections in the central nervous system. Also known by the French term tic douleureux (painful twitch), as the short-lived episodes of pain in this disorder are so severe as to cause patients to wince.

Vertebra (plural: vertebrae): a bone of the spine, composed of, in part, the vertebral body, lamina, and facets.

Vertebral bodies: the supporting part of a vertebra in the front of the spine, which takes the greatest weight. The disks are located between the vertebral bodies.

Vertebroplasty: a technique in which liquified orthopedic bone cement is injected into partially collapsed pain-generating bones (usually vertebral bodies) with the intent of relieving otherwise poorly controlled pain. This therapy is especially beneficial in patients suffering from painful vertebral fractures caused by osteoporosis or cancer.

Visceral pain: pain arising from the internal organs or viscera.

Yellow ligament: see *ligamentum flavum.*

RESOURCES

Inquire directly to department chairmen or directors of the services to obtain information and the names of physicians specializing in your problem.

Medical Centers Specializing in Pain, State by State

These pain-management programs are usually staffed by anesthesiologists, unless otherwise indicated. Self-referral to these programs is primarily to gain pain relief, including through the use of narcotics. Many of those listed tend to rely heavily on blocks to alleviate pain. These programs vary greatly in their ability to diagnose the source of pain and to refer patients for the best radiological studies or surgery when needed. They can also differ greatly in their expertise in using implantable technologies (spinal-cord stimulation, implantable pumps), radiofrequency lesions (especially in the neck or thoracic spine), and destructive lesions for cancer pain. Some of these centers may not perform discography or other procedures for treating discogenic pain. Most of these centers do not perform vertebroplasty.

The list below is not comprehensive, nor does inclusion in the list constitute an endorsement of a program. At the same time, omission from these pages does not imply a poor opinion of a physician or a pain-management program.

ARIZONA
The University of Arizona Health
  Science Center
Pain Management Services
1501 N. Campbell Ave.
P.O. Box 245114
Tucson, AZ 85724-5114
Phone: 520-626-5119
Fax: 520-626-3007
Medical Director, Pain Program:
  Bennet E. Davis, M.D.
E-mail: bdavis@u.arizona.edu

CALIFORNIA
University of California at Davis
  Medical Center
2315 Stockton Blvd.
Sacramento, CA 95817
Phone: 916-734-6824
Fax: 916-734-6826
Medical Director, Pain Program:
  Scott Fishman, M.D.

University of California at
  San Francisco
Pain Management Center
2255 Post St.
San Francisco, CA 94143-1654
Phone: 415-885-7246
Fax: 415-885-3883
Medical Director, Pain Program:
  Pamela Palmer, M.D.

Stanford University
Pain Management Center
A-408 Boswell Building
300 Pasteur Dr.
Stanford, CA 94305
Phone: 650-723-6238
Fax: 650-725-7743
Director, Pain Management Program:
  Raymond R. Gaeta, M.D.
E-mail: gaeta@leland.stanford.edu

COLORADO
University of Colorado Health
  Science Center
Pain Management Center
4701 E. 9th Ave.

Denver, CO 80262
Phone: 303-372-8100
Fax: 303-372-7659
Director, Pain Management Program:
  Jose M. Angel, M.D.

CONNECTICUT
Lloyd Saberski, M.D. (Internist,
  anesthesiologist, and
  interventional pain
  specialist)
Medical staff, attending physician,
  Yale New Haven Hospital
Office:
40 Temple St., Suite 4D
New Haven, CT 06520-8073
Phone: 203-624-4208

FLORIDA
Mayo Clinic Jacksonville
4500 San Pablo Rd.
Jacksonville, FL 32224
Phone: 904-296-5288
Fax: 904-296-3877
Director, Pain Management Program:
  Tim Lamer, M.D.
  (anesthesiologist)
E-mail: marshall.Kenneth@mayo.edu

University of Miami
Jackson Memorial Medical Center
1611 NW 12th Ave.
Miami, FL 33136
Phone: 305-585-6283
Fax: 305-545-6753
Director, Pain Management Program:
  Fred Furgang, M.D.
  (anesthesiologist)

GEORGIA
The Emory Clinic
Center for Pain Management
1364 Clifton Rd, NE
Atlanta, GA 30322
Phone: 404-778-5582
Fax: 404-778-3952
Director, Division of Pain Medicine:
  Allen Hord, M.D.
E-mail: allen_hord@emory.org

ILLINOIS
Northwestern Anesthesiology and
    Pain Medicine
675 North St. Clair St.
Galter Pavilion, Suite 20-100
Chicago, IL 60611
Phone: 312-695-2500
Fax: 312-695-7605
Medical Director, Pain Program:
    Honorio T. Benzon, M.D.

IOWA
University of Iowa
Department of Anesthesia
200 Hawkins Dr.
Iowa City, IA 52242-1079
Phone: 319-356-2633
Fax: 319-356-2940
Medical Director: Richard W.
    Rosenquist, M.D.

MARYLAND
Johns Hopkins Pain Center
601 N. Caroline Street, Suite 3062
Baltimore, MD 21287
Phone: 410-955-PAIN
Fax: 410-614-2993
Medical Director: Peter Staats, M.D.
    (neurologist)
Department of Neurosurgery:
    Richard North, M.D.
    (specialist in lumbar-spinal-cord
    stimulation, implantable
    intraspinal pumps, nerve blocks,
    lumbar radiofrequency-lesioning
    procedures for facet pain)

MASSACHUSETTS
Beth Israel Deaconess Medical
    Center, Harvard Medical School
330 Brookline Ave.
Boston, MA 02215
Phone: 617-667-3334
Fax: 617-754-2677
Director, Pain Management Program:
    Christine Peegers-Asdourian, M.D.

Brigham and Women's Hospital
Pain Management Center

75 Francis St.
Boston, MA 02115
Phone: 617-732-6708
Fax: 617-731-5953
Director: Edgar L. Ross, M.D.
E-mail: ross@zeus.bwh.harvard.edu

Massachusetts General Hospital
Pain Center
15 Parkman St., WACC 324
Boston, MA 02114-3139
Phone: 617-726-8810
Fax: 617-724-2719
Director, Pain Center:
    Jane Ballantyne, M.D.
    (anesthesiologist)
Department of Neurosurgery: Ernest
    Mathews, M.D. (trigeminal
    neuralgia and spinal disorders)
Director, Head and Neck Pain
    Center: Martin Acquadro, M.D.

New England Medical Center
Tufts University Department of
    Anesthesia
Box 298
750 Washington St.
Boston, MA 02111
Phone: 617-636-6208 or 6044
Fax: 617-636-4674
Director, Pain Management Program:
    Andrew W. Sukiennik, M.D.

MINNESOTA
Mayo Clinic
200 First St. SW
Rochester, MN 55905
Phone: 507-284-9694
Fax: 507-284-0120
Director, Pain Division; Chairman,
    Department of Anesthesia: David
    P. Martin, M.D.

NEW HAMPSHIRE
Dartmouth Hitchcock Medical Center
Medical Center Dr.
Lebanon, NH 03756
Phone: 603-650-8391
Fax: 603-650-8199

Medical Director, Pain Program:
  Gilbert Fanciullo, M.D.
E-mail:
  leana.wiechnik@hitchcock.org

NEW MEXICO
University of New Mexico School of
  Medicine
Department of Anesthesia, Surge
  Bldg.
2701 Frontier St., NE
Albuquerque, NM 87131-5216
Phone: 505-272-2610
Fax: 505-272-1300
Department Chairman: Stephen E.
  Abram, M.D.
E-mail: sabram@salud.unm.edu

NEW YORK
Albany Medical Center, Anesthesia
  A-131
47 New Scotland Ave.
Albany, NY 12208
Phone: 888-590-PAIN
Fax: 518-262-4736
Director, Pain Clinic: Eugene Lucier,
  M.D.

Beth Israel Medical Center
Department of Pain and Palliative
  Care
First Ave. at 16th St.
New York, NY 10003
Chairman: Russell Portenoy, M.D.
Phone: 212-844-1505
Fax: 212-844-1503

Mount Sinai Pain Management
  Service
5 E. 98th St., 6th floor
New York, NY 10029
Phone: 212-241-6372
Director: Joel Kreitzer, M.D.

Cornell University Medical College
The New York Hospital
525 E. 68th St.
New York, NY 10021
Phone: 212-746-2960

Fax: 212-746-2023
Director, Pain Management Program:
  Sudhir Diwan, M.D.

New York University Medical
  Center
Department of Anesthesiology
Pain Management Center
530 First Ave.
New York, NY 10016
Phone: 212-263-7316
Fax: 212-263-7901
Director: Michel Dubois, M.D.

New York University Medical Center
Departments of Neurology and
  Radiology
530 First Ave., Suite 5A
New York, NY 10016
Phone: 212-263-6123
Fax: 212-263-6878
Emile Hiesiger, M.D.
  (pharmacological pain
  management and interventional,
  pain-relieving procedures)
Email: doctor@hiesiger.com
Web site: www.hiesiger.com

Memorial Sloan-Kettering Cancer
  Center
Pain Service Department
1275 York Ave.
New York, NY 10021
Phone: 212-639-6851
Fax: 212-717-3206
Director, Pain Management
  Program: Subhash Jain, M.D.
  (anesthesiologist)
Chief, Pain and Palliative Service:
  Richard Payne, M.D. (neurologist)

Manhattan Center for Pain
  Management
St. Luke's-Roosevelt Hospital
1000 Tenth Ave.
New York, NY 10019
Phone: 212-523-6357
Director, Pain Management Service:
  Ronald Hertz, M.D.

Columbia Presbyterian Medical
Center for Oral, Facial and Head
Pain
Harkness Pavilion 806
630 W. 168th St.
New York, NY 10032
Phone: 212-305-2571
Steven J. Scrivani, D.D.S., M.D. (for
oral, facial, and head pain)
Email: sus4@columbia.edu

NORTH CAROLINA
Duke Pain and Palliative Care
Program
Duke University Medical Center
P.O. Box 2964
Durham, NC 27710
Phone: 919-681-2272
Fax: 919-681-7094
Medical Director: Shashidhar H.
Kori, M.D. (neurologist)

OHIO
Cleveland Clinic Foundation Pain
Management Center
9500 Euclid Ave., U21
Cleveland, OH 44195
Phone: 216-444-2674
Fax: 216-444-0797
Director, Pain Management Center
and Program: Nagy A. Mekhail,
M.D., Ph.D.
E-mail: omabegb@cesmtp.ccf.org

OREGON
Oregon Health Science University
3181 SW Sam Jackson Park Rd.,
UHS-2
Portland, OR 97201
Phone: 503-494-5370
Fax: 503-494-7635
Director, Pain Management Program:
Brett Stacey, M.D.
(anesthesiologist)
E-mail: staceyb@ohsu.edu

Good Samaritan Hospital
Department of Neurology and
Neurosurgery

1040 N.W. 22nd Ave., Suite NSC-
460
Portland, OR 97210
Phone: 503-413-7293
José Ochoa, D.S.C., M.D., Ph.D.
(special interest in neuropathic pain
and CRPS)

PENNSYLVANIA
Jefferson University Physicians,
Department of Neurosurgery
1015 Chestnut St., Suite 1400
Philadelphia, PA 19107
Phone: 215-955-6744
Giancarlo Barolat, M.D. (cervical
and lumbar spinal-cord
stimulation)

Matthew T. Kline, M.D. (pain
management, including nerve blocks
and radiofrequency lesioning)
Affiliated with Elkins Park Hospital
and Abington Surgery Center
1010 Fox Chase Rd.
Rockledge, PA 19046
Phone: 215-663-8585
Fax: 215-663-8447

University of Pennsylvania Health
System, Presbyterian Medical
Center
Suite 140
Medical Office Building
39th and Market Sts.
Philadelphia, PA 19104-2699
Phone: 215-662-8650
Fax: 215-349-4616
Director, Pain Medicine Center:
F. Michael Ferrante, M.D.

SOUTH CAROLINA
Medical University of South
Carolina
171 Ashley Ave.
Charleston, SC 29425-2207
Phone: 843-792-2322
Fax: 843-792-2726
Director, Pain Management Program:
Jeffrey W. Folk, M.D.

TENNESSEE
Vanderbilt University Pain Control
  Center
1211 21st Ave. South
Medical Arts Building, Suite 401
Nashville, TN 37232-4125
Phone: 615-936-1201
Fax: 615-936-1313
Director, Pain Fellowship Program:
  Benjamin W. Johnson, Jr., M.D.,
  M.B.A., DABPM, CIME

TEXAS
University of Texas M. D. Anderson
  Cancer Center
Symptom Control and Palliative Care
  Program
Box 8, 1515 Holcombe Blvd.
Houston, TX 77030
Phone: 713-792-6085
Fax: 713-794-6092
Clinic Medical Director: Larry
  Driver, M.D. (anesthesiologist)

Texas Tech University Pain
  Management Clinic
Health Sciences Center
3601 4th St., 1C282
Lubbock, TX 79430
Phone: 806-743-3112
Fax: 806-742-2984
Director: Gabor Racz, M.D.
  (anesthesiologist)

UTAH
University of Utah Health Sciences
  Center
Pain Management Center
546 Chipeta Way, Suite 2000
Salt Lake City, UT 84108
Phone: 801-585-7690
Fax: 801-585-7694
Director, Pain Medicine Program:
  Michael A. Asburn, M.D., M.P.H.

VIRGINIA
University of Virginia Health Science
  Center
Department of Anesthesiology

P.O. Box 800710
Charlottesville, VA 22908
Phone: 804-924-2283
Fax: 804-982-0019
Medical Director, Pain Program:
  Robin J. Hamill-Ruth, M.D.

WASHINGTON
Pain Center at Roosevelt Clinic
4245 Roosevelt Way NE
Seattle, WA 98105-6920
Phone: 206-598-4282
John Loeser, M.D. (neurosurgery)

Professional Associations Dedicated to Pain Management

American Academy of Head, Neck
  and Facial Pain
520 West Pipeline Rd.
Hurst, TX 76053
Phone: 800-322-8651
Web site: www.aahnfp.org

American Academy of Orofacial
  Pain
19 Mantua Rd.
Mount Royal, NJ 08061
Phone: 856-423-3629
Fax: 856-423-3420
E-mail: aaohq@talley.com
Web site: www.aaop.org

American Academy of Pain
  Management
13947 Mono Way #A
Sonora, CA 95370
Phone: 209-533-9744
Fax: 209-533-9750
E-mail: aapm@aapainmanage.org
Web site: www.aapainmanage.org

American Association for the Study
  of Headache
19 Mantua Rd.
Mount Royal, NJ 08061
Phone: 856-423-0043
Fax: 856-423-0082
E-mail: aashhq@talley.com
Web site: www.aash.org

American Chronic Pain Association
P.O. Box 850
Rocklin, CA 95677-0850
Phone: 916-632-0922
Fax: 916-632-3208
Web site: www.theacpa.org

American Council for Headache
  Education
19 Mantua Rd.
Mount Royal, NJ 08061
Phone: 856-423-0258 or
  1-800-255-2243
Fax: 856-423-0082
E-mail: aashhq@talley.com
Web site: www.achenet.org

American Pain Foundation
111 South Calvert St., Suite 2700
Baltimore, MD 21202
Web site: www.painfoundation.org

American Society for Addition
  Medicine
4601 North Park Ave., Arcade Suite
  101
Chevy Chase, MD 20815
Phone: 301-656-3920
Fax: 301-656-3815
E-mail: Email@asam.org
Web site: www.asam.org

American Society of Law, Medicine
  and Ethics
Phone: 617-262-4990
Fax: 617-437-7596
Web site: www.aslme.org

Arthritis Foundation
1330 W. Peachtree St.
Atlanta, GA 30309
Phone: 404-872-7100 or
  1-800-283-7800
E-mail: help@arthritis.org
Web site: www.arthritis.org

Back Pain Association of America
P.O. Box 135
Pasadena, MD 21122-0135

Phone: 410-255-3633
Fax: 410-255-7338
E-mail: backpainassoc@Fmsn.com

Cancer Care, Inc.
275 Seventh Ave., 22nd floor
New York, NY 10001
Phone: 212-221-3300 or
  1-800-813-4673
E-mail: info@cancercare.org
Web site: www.cancercareinc.org

Candlelighters Childhood Cancer (for
  families of childhood cancer suffer-
  ers, survivors of childhood cancer,
  and their professional caretakers)
7910 Woodmont Ave., Suite 460
Bethesda, MD 20814-3015
Phone: 1-800-366-2223
Fax: 301-718-2686
E-mail: info@candlelighters.org
Web site: www.candlelights.org

International Association for the
  Study of Pain
Louisa E. Jones, Executive Officer
909 NE 43rd St., Suite 306
Seattle, WA 98105-6020
Phone: 206-547-6409
Fax: 206-547-1703
Web site: www.halcyon.com/iasp

Interstitial Cystitis Association
51 Monroe St., Suite 1402
Rockville, MD 20850
Phone: 301-610-5300 or
  1-800-HELP-ICA
Fax: 301-610-5308
Web site: www.ichelp.com

JAMA Migraine Information Center
American Medical Association
Web site: www.ama-assn.org/special/
  migraine/newsline/newsline.htm

Last Acts Web Site (dedicated to
  improving care at the end of a
  person's life)
Web site: www.lastacts.org

National Association for the
  Treatment of Pain
1330 Skyline Dr., #21
Monterey, CA 93940
Phone: 831-655-8812
Fax: 831-655-2823
Web site: www.paincare.org

National Chronic Pain Outreach
  Association
P.O. Box 274
Milboro, VA 24460
Phone: 540-862-9437

National Headache Foundation
428 W. St. James Pl., 2nd floor
Chicago, IL 60614
Phone: 773-388-6399 or
  1-800-843-2256
Fax: 312-525-7357
Web site: www.headaches.org

National Multiple Sclerosis
  Association
733 Third Ave.
New York, NY 10017-3288
Phone: 800-344-4867
Fax: 212-986-7981
E-mail: info@nmss.org
Web site: www.mnss.org

National Vulvodynia Association
Executive Director: Phyllis Mate
P.O. Box 4491
Silver Spring, MD 20914-4491
Phone: 301-299-0775
Fax: 301-299-3999
Web site: www.nva.org

Neuropathy Association
60 E. 42nd St., Suite 942
New York, NY 10165
Phone: 212-692-0662
Fax: 212-692-0068
Web site: www.neuropathy.org

Pain & Policy Studies Group (focuses
  on drug regulation)
University of Wisconsin–Madison
1900 University Ave.
Madison, WI 53705
Phone: 608-263-7662
Fax: 608-263-0259
Web site:
  www.medsch.wisc.edu/painpolicy/

Reflex Sympathetic Dystrophy
  Syndrome Association
P.O. Box 821
Haddonfield, NJ 08033
Phone: 609-795-8845
Fax: 856-795-8845
Web site: www.rsds.org

TMJ Association, Ltd. (for
  temporomandibular-joint pain)
5418 W. Washington Blvd.
Milwaukee, WI 53212
Phone: 414-259-3223
Fax: 414-259-8112
E-mail: info@tmj.org

Trigeminal Neuralgia Association
P.O. Box 340
Barnegat Light, NJ 08006
Phone: 609-361-1014
Fax: 609-361-0982
Web site: neurosurgery.mgh.harvard.
  edu/tna/

VZV Research Foundation (for
  shingles)
40 E. 72nd St., Room 4B
New York, NY 10021
Phone: 212-472-3181 or
  1-800-472-8478
Web site:
  vzvfoundation.org/index.cfm

SUGGESTED READING

Byock, Ira, M.D. *Dying Well: Peace and Possibilities at the End of Life.* New York: Riverhead Books, 1998.

Caudill, Margaret A., M.D., Ph.D. *Managing Pain Before It Manages You.* New York: Guilford Press, 1999.

Fishman, Loren, and Carol Ardman. *Back Pain: How to Relieve Low Back Pain and Sciatica.* New York: W. W. Norton, 1999.

Fishman, Scott, M.D., with Lisa Berger. *The War on Pain.* New York: Harper-Collins, 2000.

Kabat-Zinn, Jon. *Wherever You Go. There You Are: Mindfulness Meditation in Everyday Life.* New York: Hyperion, 1995.

Kübler-Ross, Elisabeth, M.D. *On Death and Dying.* New York: Collier Books, 1997.

Lang, Susan S., and Richard B. Patt, M.D. *You Don't Have to Suffer: A Complete Guide to Relieving Cancer Pain for Patients and Their Families,* New York: Oxford University Press, 1995.

Livingston, William K., and Howard L. Fields. *Pain and Suffering.* Seattle: International Association for the Study of Pain, 1998.

Morris, David B. *The Culture of Pain.* Berkeley: University of California Press, 1993.

———. *Illness and Culture.* Berkeley: University of California Press, 1998.

Nuland, Sherwin B. *How We Die: Reflections on Life's Final Chapter.* New York: Vintage Books, 1995.

Ramachandran, V. S., and Sandra Blakeslee. *Phantoms in the Brain: Probing the Mysteries of the Human Mind.* New York: Quill, 1999.

Rapaport, Alan M., M.D., and Fred D. Sheftell, M.D. *Headache Relief: A Comprehensive, Up-to-Date, Medically Proven Program That Can Control and Ease Headache Pain.* New York: Fireside, 1991.

————. *Headache Relief for Women: How You Can Manage and Prevent Pain.* New York: Little, Brown & Company, 1996.

Sadler, Jan, with Patrick Wall. *Natural Pain Relief: A Practical Handbook for Self-Help.* New York: Element, 1997.

Sarno, John E. *Healing Back Pain: The Mind-Body Connection.* New York: Warner Books, 1991.

INDEX

Page numbers in *italics* refer to illustrations.

abdomen, 2, 19, 30
abdominal cancers, 2
abortion, 178
acetaminophen (Tylenol), xvi, 40, 42,
  57, 71, 93, 140, 170
Achilles tendon, 19
ACL (anterior cruciate ligament)
  injuries, 164–66
acne, 44
acupuncture, xvi, 30, 34–35, 38, 69,
  87, 117
acute pain, 2–3
addiction, fear of, *see* narcotics, fear of
  addiction to
Advil (ibuprofen), 24, 42–43, 175
AIDS, 43, 45
  neuropathic pain of, 139–41, 213
  treatment of, 140–41
aladronate (Fosamax), 97
alcohol, 67
  interaction of medication with, 24, 42
  in moderation, 22
  travel and, 24

Aleve (naproxen), 24, 43
alternative medicine, xvi, 26, 33–38
  acupuncture, xvi, 30, 34–35, 38, 69,
    87, 116
  effectiveness of, 33–34, 38
  laser energy to the skin, 35
  potential harm of, 34
  spinal manipulation, 33, 35–38, 85
  studies of, 33
American Academy of Pain Medicine, 55
American Geriatric Society, 61
*American Journal of Obstetrics and
  Gynecology,* 176–77
American Pain Society, 55, 202
American Society of Anesthesiologists,
  34
amitriptyline (Elavil), 45, 46
amphetamines, 56
analgesics, 26, 36
anesthesia, 34, 41
anesthesia dolorosa, 134
angina, 13
Anglo-Saxon Protestants, 11

animals, 10–11
ankles:
    sprained, 10, 159
    spread of pain to, 12
anterior cruciate ligament (ACL)
    injuries, 164–66
antiarrhythmics, 48
anticancer drugs, 94, 191–98
anticonvulsants, 42, 46–48, 69, 136,
    139, 143
antidepressants, 41, 45–46, 57, 80
    selective serotonin receptor
        inhibitors, 46
    tricyclic, 45–46, 58, 69, 76, 136,
        138–39
anxiety, 3, 4, 9, 10, 31–32, 46, 76, 86
arachnoiditis, 149–50
Aridea (pamindronate), 97
arm pain, 12, 13, 22, 27
arthritis, 37, 41, 91, 92
    osteoarthritis, 50, 92–94
    pain of, 2, 35, 41, 73, 85
    treatment of, 42, 43, 44, 92–95
    see also rheumatoid arthritis
aspartate, 8, 49
aspirin, 2, 24, 40, 41, 42, 71
asthma, xvi, 40, 43
atherosclerosis, 25, 138
athletics, 20–22, 92
    competitive, 21
    moderation in, 21
    potentially dangerous, 21
    preventing injuries in, 21
    reducing performance level in, 21
    weekend, 19, 21
    see also exercise; sports injuries
automobile accidents, 2, 130, 217
axon, 5, 49, 50, 52
azothiaprine (Imuran), 94

back:
    injuries of, 20
    relaxing of, 19
    sleeping on, 20
backpacks, 20
back pain, 2, 14, 18, 101–28
    diagnostic challenge of, 114–16
    key points about, 128
    low, 22, 24, 35–37, 91, 109–11, 117
    prevention of, 19, 22–23
    treatment of, 35–37, 42, 115–28
    wear and tear as cause of, 104–6
    see also specific conditions
baclofen (Lioresal), 48, 133

behavioral therapy, 26, 28, 31, 32
Bellevue Hospital, 11
Benjamin, Vallo, v
Benson, Herbert, 27
beta blockers, 69
bicipital tendinitis, 162
biofeedback, 28–29, 38, 69, 71, 92, 148
birth control pill, 37, 67
bladder, 4, 104
    problems of, 30, 91, 109, 125, 174
bleeding, 43
    control of, 8, 171
blood:
    clotting mechanism of, 43
    insufficient supply of, 30, 37
blood pressure, 28
    control of, 70
    elevation of, 2, 5, 40
    high, xvi, 25
    lowering of, 27, 200
blood tests, 15
blood vessels, 4
    abnormal dilation of, 65, 67, 68, 70,
        131
    expansion and leakage of, 50
    hardening and clogging of, 25, 138
body:
    nighttime positioning of, 20
    at play, 20–22
    as your instrument, 19
bone-density tests, 100
bones:
    disintegration of, 95–100
    fractures of, 2
    mending of, xv
    tumors invading, 3
    see also osteoporosis
Bonica, John, 219
Botox (botulinum toxin) injections,
    68–69, 88
brain, 11
    blocking pain message to, xv, 3
    damage of, 78
    emotional area of, 5, 6
    growth of, 12–13
    lesions of, 199
    modulation of pain message to, 5–9,
        8, 41, 45
    sensory processing area of, 5, 6,
        131–32
    testing function in, 15
    transmission of pain message to, 4–8,
        6, 8–9, 8, 12, 13, 31–32
    tumors of, 44, 131

brain-wave activity, 27, 28
breast cancer, 97, 186, 188, 199
buproprion (Welbutrin), 46
burners and stingers, 169
burns, 2–3, 9
bursitis, 19, 34, 109

caffeine, 68, 71
Calcimar (salmon calcitonin), 97
calcium, 96, 97
calcium channel blockers, 70
calisthenics, 18
cancer, xv, 184–203
    body's response to pain medication
        for, 198
    pain management and, 201–3
    treatment of, 95, 186, 189–97
    see also specific cancers
cancer pain, xv, 1, 2, 184–203
    key points about, 203
    treatment of, 30, 45, 55
capsaicin (Zostrix), 49–50, 139
carbamazepine (Tegretol), 47, 132–33,
        139, 154
cardiologists, xvi
carotid arteries, 70
cartilage, 92, 93
Catapress (clonidine), 145
CAT scan, 14, 73, 77, 98, 107, 113,
        114, 150
cauda equina (horse's tail), 6, 104, 105,
        106, 112, 125
Celebrex, 43–44
Central Florida Health Care Coalition,
        221
cerebral palsy, 127, 133
Cervantes, Miguel de, 64
cervical cancer, 43
cervical collar, 22, 117
cervical radiofrequency facet
        neurotomy, 74–75
chairs, 20, 22
    kneeler, 20
    straight-backed, 20
chemical hypophysectomy, 199
chemicals:
    body, 8
    irritation with, 5
chemical sympathectomy, 144–45
chemotherapy, 45, 192
childbirth, 2, 9, 10
children, 10
    carrying of, 19
    hyperactive, 12

Chinese, 11
chiropractors, 33, 35–38, 85
chlamydia, 178
chronic pain:
    acute flare-ups with, 2
    as a black cloud, 3
    challenge of, 3, 41–42
    chronic undertreatment of, 3–4,
        39–40
    controllable vs. uncontrollable, xv
    determining individual reactions to,
        xv
    difficulty in finding causes of, 1–2,
        3–4, 13–15, 40
    emotional response to, xv, 3, 31–32,
        131
    extension beyond original site of, 2,
        11, 12–13
    family impact of, xv, 131
    human suffering and, xiii, xv, xvi, 3
    "learn to live with it" approach to, xv
    long-lived duration of, xv, 2, 13
    lost wages and work associated with,
        xiii, 4, 42, 65
    number of Americans affected by,
        xiii, xv, 3
    obtaining good health care for,
        xiii–xvii, 204–18
    permanent disability stemming from,
        4, 42
    psychological pain resulting from, 3,
        4, 10, 131
    psychological problems blamed for,
        3, 13, 83, 130
    quality of life affected by, xv, 3, 4, 221
    secondary psychiatric symptoms
        stemming from, 15, 131
    survival value lacking in, 3
    uncovering mysteries of, 1–16
    worsening of, 13
    see also pain
chronic pelvic pain without obvious
        pathology (CPPWOP), 174–75
cingulumotomy, 199
cisplatinum, 192
Civil War, U.S., 141
clonazepam (Klonopin), 47–48, 78,
        133, 148
clonidine (Catapress), 145
cocaine, 37, 54
coccydynia, 113
coccyx, 101, 102, 103, 113–14
codeine, 56, 140
cold, 5

cold packs, 87
colon cancer, 197
complementary medicine, xvi, 26, 33–38
    see also alternative medicine
complex regional pain syndrome
        (CRPS), 11, 12, 141–46
    oral drug therapy for, 144–45
    pain management of, 143–44
    symptoms of, 142–43
    Type I, 141, 145
    Type II, 142
constipation, 24, 33, 42, 51, 56, 61
cortex, 9, 67
    stimulation of, 156–57
corticosteroids, 44, 68, 94, 119, 143,
        192–93
coughing, 24
COX-2 inhibitor drugs, 43–44
cringing, 10
cryoanalgesia, 122, 136, 198, 200
cyclo-oxygenase (COX), 43

Danocrine (danazol), 178
Dart, Maryann, 142
decongestants, 37
dementia pugilistica, 78
Demerol (meperidine), 54, 130
dendrites, 5, 52
Depakote (valproic acid), 47, 48, 69,
        133
depression, 3, 4, 10, 31, 32, 44, 45, 46,
        69, 76, 86, 131, 199
desipramine (Norpramin), 45, 46, 138
dextromethorphan, 48–49
diabetes, 137–39, 153–54
    pain associated with, 14, 45
diabetic neuropathy, 137–39, 186
diagnosis, xiii, 3, 15
    key points of, 16
    tests for, xvi, 14
Dickinson, Emily, 1
digestive system disturbances, 25, 43
dihydroergotamine (DHE-45), 68
Dilantin (phenytoin), 47, 133, 139
Dilaudid (hydromorphinone), 51, 54,
        56, 57
dimethylsulfoxide (DMSO), 180–81
discogenic pain, description of, 107
discography, 107, 124, 212
disks, 13, 18, 101–6, 102
    damaged and diseased, 15, 22,
        104–6, 112
    nerve compression in, 14, 22, 24,
        107–9

pain in, 24, 106, 107
    see also herniated disks
distal symmetrical polyneuropathies
        (DSPN), 139–40
dizziness, 80
dorsal root entry zone, 6
dreams, 45
DREZ lesion, 155
Duragesic (fentanyl), 51, 54, 56, 58
dyspareunia, 182–83

earaches, 132
ears, 4
Effexor (venlaxafine), 46
Elavil (amitriptyline), 45, 46
electromyography (EMG), 114–15,
        119, 169
Embrel (etanercept), 95
emergency rooms, 11, 130
Emla Cream (lidocaine and prilocaine),
        49
emphysema, 61
endocrinologists, 97, 213
endometriosis, 176–78
endorphins, 8, 51, 53
epidural steroid injections, 44, 118,
        124
epiduroscopy, 118–19
epilepsy, 42
ergonomic furniture, 18, 92
ergotamine drugs, 68, 70
esophagitis, 44
esophagus, 25, 107
estrogen, 96, 179
estrogen replacement, 97
etanercept (Embrel), 95
Evista (raloxifene hydrochloride), 97
exercise, xvi
    common sense rules of, 19–20
    cooling down after, 21
    moderation in, 19, 21
    preventing injuries in, 19, 21
    programs of, 19, 21, 37
    starting slowly with, 21
    warming up before, 18, 19, 21, 86
    weight-bearing, 97
Exorcist, The, 104
eyebrow pain, 14
eyes, 4, 134

facet blocks, 119
facet joints, 13, 14, 20, 74–75, 98,
        103, 105
    pain in, 15, 106–7

facial pain, 14, 30, 46–47, 64, 131
  atypical, 75–76
fanny belts, 23
fentanyl (Duragesic), 51, 54, 56, 58
fibroids, 179
fibromyalgia, 86, 90–92
  pain and soreness of, 2, 11, 12,
    90–91, 220
  treatment of, 45, 92
fibrosis, 174
fight-or-flight response, 27
financial problems, 4, 32
Fioricet (caffeine, butalbital, and
    acetaminophen), 71, 72
Fiorinal (caffeine, butalbital, and
    aspirin), 71
fire, 2–3
fluoxetine (Prozac), 46, 69
Food and Drug Administration, U.S.
    (FDA), 35, 178, 180
foot ulcers, 138
foramen, 103, 104, 112
foramenotomy, 126
forehead:
  pain impulses from, 13
  water torture on, 1, 12
Fosamax (aladronate), 97
fractures:
  osteoporotic, 27, 95, 112, 186
  stress, 163–64
  see also specific fractures

GABA, 8, 47–48
gabapentin (Neurontin), 47, 48, 69,
    133, 136, 139, 140
gardening, 19
gastric cancer, 99
gastritis, 43, 44
gastroenterologists, 33
glaucoma, 46, 138
glucosamine, 33, 93
glutamate, 8, 49
glycerol injections, 133–34
grimaces, 10, 96
gymnastics, 21
gynecologic pain, 173–83
  key points about, 183
  see also specific conditions

hair shirts, xvi
head:
  pain in, 14, 30, 37, 84
  trauma to, 78–84
headaches, xvi, 2, 4, 14, 30, 64–84

cervicogenic, 72–73
cluster, 69–71
key points about, 84
migraine, 28, 65–69, 72, 169–70
possible causes of, 64–65, 67, 70,
    71–72, 76–84
post-traumatic, 72–73
rebound, 71–72
sports, 169–70
tension, 1, 28–29, 69, 71, 72, 170
treatment of, 35, 41, 42, 67–69,
    70–72, 73–75
headache specialists, 69, 73–74, 84
Health and Human Services
    Department, U.S., Agency for
    Health Care Policy and Research
    of, 36
health-care professionals, xiii–xiv
  key points about, 218
  obtaining good care from, xiii–xvii,
    204–18
  working as an educated partner with,
    xiii–xiv, 205–7, 216–18
  see also physicians; specific medical
    specialties
health maintenance organizations
    (HMOs), 205, 206, 208
heart:
  pain in, 13
  risks to, of excess weight, 25
heart attacks, 25
  death from, 13
  referred pain in, 13
heartbeat, 5, 28
heart failure, 25, 43
heart rate, increase in, 5
heart-rhythm disturbances, 46
heat, 5
  testing reaction to, 10–11
herbal remedies, 33, 34
herniated disks, 15, 37, 89, 107–9, 166
  cause of, 19, 20, 25
  cervical, 19, 20, 27, 108, 109, 117
  lumbar, 107–8, 109, 117, 129
  sciatica stemming from, 111
  thoracic, 109
  treatment of, 26, 45, 115–18,
    124–27
heroin, 54
high blood pressure, xvi, 25
hips:
  artificial, 25, 44
  fracture of, 39
HIV, 139–41, 147

HMOs (health maintenance
    organizations), 205, 206, 208
Hodgkin's disease, 191, 192
hormones, 96, 97, 176
horseback riding, 21, 166
horse's tail (cauda equina), 6, 104, *105*,
    106, *112*, 125
hospitals, xvii, 39, 96
howling, 11
Hugo, Victor, 101
Huxley, Thomas Henry, 39
Hyalen (sodium hyaluronate), 93
hydromorphinone (Dilaudid), 51, 54,
    56, 57
hydroxychloroquine (Plaquenil), 94
hyperactivity, 12
hypnosis, 28, 29, 38, 148
hypothalamus, 199
hysterectomy, 2

ibuprofen (Advil; Motrin), 24, 42–43,
    175
ice packs, xvi, 165
iliotibial-band syndrome, 162
imagining techniques, 13–14, 15, 16
imipramine (Tofranil), 45
Imitrex (sumatriptan), 68, 70
immune system, 44
impotence, 25
Imuran (azothiaprine), 94
Inderal, 69
India, 18
Indocin (indomethacin), 70
insurance companies, xvii, 2
International Association for the Study
    of Pain (IASP), 141
interstitial cystitis, 180–81
intestinal problems, 2
intradiscal electrothermal lysis (IDET),
    121–22
intradiscal radiofrequency lesioning,
    120
intravenous regional sympathetic
    blockade, 144
Irish, 11
irritable bowel disease, 91
isotope-based positron emission
    tomography (PET scan), 15
Italians, 11

jaws, 2, 30, 45, 76–78
Jefferson, Thomas, 219
Jews, 11
Johnson, Samuel, 204

joints, 4, 18, 42, 159
    artificial, 25, 93–94
    drug treatment for pain in, 92–93
Jones, Franklin, 123–24
Jones, Maggie, 152
*Journal of the American Medical
    Association,* 33
Judeo-Christian tradition, xvi
Jung, Carl, 85

Kaposi's sarcoma, 192
Kennedy, John F., 21, 86
Kevorkian, Jack, 197
kidney disease, 25
kidneys, 43, 188
Klonopin (clonazepam), 47–48, 78,
    133, 148
knees, 162
    arthritic, 41, 92
    artificial, 25, 26
    injuries of, 164–66

laboratory tests, 16
Lachman's test, 165
laminectomy, 116, 126
laser treatment, 121–22, 181
legs:
    fractures of, 2, 40, 54
    pain in, 12, 129, 130
    poor circulation in, 137–38
leprosy, 137
lesioning procedures, 198–201
leukemia, 191
lidocaine, 49
Lidoderm (lidocaine), 49
lifestyle changes, 3, 17, 18–25, 32,
    115, 116, 176
    athletics and, 20–22
    sleeping habits and, 20
    travel and, 22–24
    weight considerations and, 19, 21,
        25
lifting, 18
    tips on, 19
ligaments, 18, 101, 106, 159
Lioresal (baclofen), 48, 133
liver, impaired function of, 42, 43, 48,
    71, 198
liver transplant, 42
Lobo, Rebecca, 164
lumbar compression fractures, 97–98
lumbar discectomy, 125–26
lumbar stenosis, 26, 37, 90, 106,
    112–13, 126

lung cancer, 186, 187–88
Lupron, 178
lupus, 91

Magic Mountain, The (Mann), xv
magnetic resonance imaging (MRI), 3,
    13–14, 15, 37, 65, 73, 77, 79, 81,
    82, 100, 107, 113, 114, 123, 131,
    222
malpractice insurance, 38
manic-depression, 70
Mann, Thomas, xv
mantras, 27
marathons, 21, 101
massage therapy, 33, 36, 37, 85, 92,
    117
mastectomies, 188
mattresses, 20
Maxalt (rizatriptan), 68
Mearns, Hughes, 129
medical histories, 3–4, 15, 16, 107
medical insurance, 38, 205–10
medical profession, xvii, 2, 3–4
medical savings accounts (MSAs), 208
medical schools, xvii
    pain curricula lacking in, 219–20
medical students, 40, 219–20
medical treatment:
    costs of, xiii, xvii, 33
    "experimental," 99
    ineffective, 33
    measuring results of, 15, 33
    progression from simplest to more
        complex forms of, xvi, 38
    range of options for, xvi
    selection of, xiii, xv, xvii
    side effects of, xiii, 33
    Western, 33, 34
Medicare, 26, 38, 99
Mediterranean diet, 22
melanoma, 43
menopause, 96, 100
menstruation, 9, 69
    irregularities of, 44, 46, 175
    pain and cramping of, 30, 43, 175,
        177
meperidine (Demerol), 54, 130
metabolic system, 25
methadone, 56
methotrexate, 94
Mexitil (mexiletine), 48, 133, 139, 148
microvascular decompression, 134
Mitchell, S. Weir, 141
modulatory procedures, 199

Montaigne, Michel de, 17
morphine, xvi, 51, 53, 54, 56, 57, 58
Motrin (ibuprofen), 24, 42–43
mountain climbing, 21, 22, 170
Mount Zion Hospital, 11
multiple sclerosis (MS), 131
muscle relaxants, 36, 71, 89
muscles, 4
    building up of, 26
    inflammation and soreness of, 11,
        12, 28, 42
    pain in, 7, 14, 85–92
    relaxation of, 27, 28–29, 36
    spasms and cramps of, 86, 88–89,
        100, 133
    strains of, 159–61
    stretching of, 18, 21, 92, 160
musculoskeletal pain, 45, 48, 85–100,
    212
    conditions associated with, 2, 11, 25,
        85–99
    deeper problems signaled by, 89–90
    key points about, 100
    treatment of, 30, 35, 87–88, 89–90,
        92–94, 95
    trigger points and, 86, 89
    see also specific conditions
Myacalcin (salmon calcitonin), 97
myofascial pain, 14, 28, 71, 80, 85–90,
    100, 186
    diagnosis of, 87
    treatment of, 87–88, 89–90
Mystery of Pain (Dickinson), 1

Naprosyn (naproxen), 24
naproxen (Aleve; Naprosyn), 24, 43
narcotics, 2, 11, 33, 39, 42, 43, 50–61,
    68, 72, 92, 130, 143, 154, 185
    around-the-clock dosage of, 60–61
    cancer treatment with, 193–97
    combining other pain medications
        with, 40, 95
    cultural views of, xvi, 40, 50
    dependence on, 54
    effective use of, 40, 42, 56–58, 93,
        95
    fear of addiction to, 40, 50–51,
        53–55
    government regulation of, 40, 50, 55
    methods of delivery with, 58–59
    physicians' unwillingness to
        prescribe, 55
    side effects of, 51–53, 55–56
    timing of, 57–58

tolerance of, 51–53
  as treatment for osteoporotic
    compression fractures, 98
National Association of Alternative
    Brokers, 208
National Institutes of Health, 33, 35,
    95
nausea, 43, 51, 56, 61, 67, 68
neck:
  extreme arching of, 19, 20
  forward-bent, 19
  injuries of, 19, 20, 22, 27, 37, 41
  pain in, 2, 14, 27, 37–38, 79–81
  surgery on, 188
nephrectomy, 188
nerve blocks, xv, 3
  diagnostic, 14, 16, 75, 77, 81–82,
    200
  treatment with, xv, 3, 119, 136–37,
    143–44
nerve conduction velocity (NCV), 114
nerve roots, compressed, 108, 110,
    111, 112
nerves:
  cranial, 131–32, 137
  damage to or dysfunction of, xv, 2,
    26, 45, 150–51, 167–69
  destruction of, 3
  electrical study of, 3
  glossopharyngeal, 132
  lesioning of, 198–201
  pressure in, 14, 26
  repeated stimulation of, 12
  scarred, 10, 45
  sympathetic, 105, 143–44
  vagus, 132
nervous system, 4–9, 6, 7, 8
  autonomic, 28, 30
  central, 4, 12–13, 34–35, 45, 52,
    91
  pain overlap in, 13–14
  peripheral, 4, 6, 12, 25, 105
  processing of pain by, 4–9, 6, 7, 8
  reducing transmission of pain to, 9
  stimulation of, 3, 6, 7, 12, 30, 34–35
Neupogen, 191
neuralgias, 2, 14, 46–47, 131–35,
    146–49
neurodystonia, 174
neurogenic claudication, 112
neurological examination, 14
neurologists, xvi, 33, 73, 74, 109, 119,
    211, 212
neuromas, 10, 45, 135–37

neurons, 5, 12, 52, 130
Neurontin (gabapentin), 47, 48, 69,
    133, 136, 139, 140
neuropathic pain, 46–47, 129–57
  black hole of, 141–43
  conditions associated with, 2, 11, 45,
    69, 131–43
  debilitating nature of, 130–31
  key points about, 157
  treatment of, 30, 45, 50, 132–35,
    136–37, 138–39, 140–41, 143–46,
    147–49, 154–55, 156–57
  see also specific conditions
neuropathies, 2, 3, 25, 37, 137–39,
    167–69
neuroscience, 4, 13
neurosurgeons, 211, 212
New England Journal of Medicine,
    139, 147–48
New York Society of Anesthesiologists,
    34
nitric oxide, 8
nonmedical pain management, 17–38
  alternative and complementary
    medicine, xvi, 26, 33–38
  biofeedback, 28–29, 38, 69, 71, 92,
    148
  hypnosis, 28, 29, 38, 148
  key points about, 38
  lifestyle changes and, 18–25
  physical therapy, xvi, 26–27, 31, 33,
    36, 38, 85, 89, 188
  psychological therapy, 28, 31–33
  relaxation response, 27, 28, 29, 33,
    38, 71, 92
  TENS, 29–31, 33, 35, 36, 87,
    116–17, 148, 154, 156, 181,
    189
nonsteroidal anti-inflammatory drugs
    (NSAIDs), 2, 36, 42–44, 57
  alcohol and, 24
  conditions treatable with, 42, 43, 68,
    71, 93, 95, 140
  deaths associated with, 43, 93
  narcotics combined with, 40
  side effects of, 24, 43, 93
  see also specific drugs
norepinephrine, 8, 45
Norpramin (desipramine), 45, 46, 38
nortriptyline (Pamelor), 45, 58, 76, 78,
    136, 138, 154
NSAIDs, see nonsteroidal
    anti-inflammatory drugs
nuclear medical techniques, 15

numbness, 22, 25, 38, 109, 129, 130, 134
nurses, 40

occupational therapy, 26
oncologists, 186–87, 202
orthopedists, 39, 211
osteoarthritis, 92–94
osteopaths, 36–37
osteoporosis, xv, 85, 95–100
    compression fractures associated with, 96, 97–99, *112*
    male, 96, 98, 99–100
    vertebroplasty treatment of, 98–100, 201
outcome analysis, v, 221–22
ovaries:
    functional cysts of, 179–80
    polycystic, 177
    removal of, 96, 100
oxycodone (Percoset), 40, 54, 56–57, 140, 192, 197

pain:
    abnormal processing of, 11–13
    aggressive treatment of, xvi
    complaints and descriptions of, xvi, 1, 2–3, 9, 10, 11, 16, 41
    controlling the disease to control, 94–95
    denial of, 24
    difficulty in measuring of, 1–2, 3–4, 14–15
    duration of, xv, 2–3
    early treatment of, xvi
    effects of personality and culture on reaction to, 9–11, 31–32
    emotional reaction to, 5, 9–10
    evaluation of, 1–2, 4, 13–16, 39–40
    gender differences and, 9
    inability to verify presence of, 1–2, 3–4, 14–15
    insufficient understanding of, 1–2
    intensity and severity of, 1, 9–11
    lancinating, 131
    learning from, 2–3, 11
    management and minimization of, xiii, xv, xvi
    memory of, 5, 9–10
    modern concepts of, xiii
    mood and, 9
    musculoskeletal, *see* musculoskeletal pain
    nonverbal expression of, 10
    perception of, 9–13, 27, 41, 199
    postoperative, 2, 10, 25, 30, 39, 187–89
    predictable, 10
    in premenopausal women, 9
    prevention of, 17, 18–25
    psychological factors and, 9
    referred, 13–14, 122–23
    short-lived duration of, 2
    subjective nature of, xvi, 1, 15
    survival value of, 2–3, 10, 11
    types of, 2–3, 9, 16, 131
    undertreatment of, xv–xvi, 2, 3–4, 39–40
    untreated, 3
    see also chronic pain
pain management teams, 201–3
pain medication, xv, xvi, 4, 11, 14, 39–63
    aging and, 61–63
    dosage and schedules of, 24, 42
    effective duration of, 24
    implanted pump delivery of, 3, 59
    inhibitory body chemicals mimicked in, 8, 41
    interaction of alcohol and, 24
    intraspinal delivery of, 58–59
    intravenous delivery of, with patient-controlled analgesia, 39, 58–59
    key points about, 63
    for painful joints, 92–93, 95
    patch delivery of, 49, 51, 56, 58, 59–60
    psychiatric, 32, 33, 45–46, 139
    side effects of, 24, 42, 47, 95
    subcutaneous delivery of, 58
    travel and, 24
    undertreatment with, 2, 39–40
    see also specific medications
pain-processing system, 4–11, *6, 7, 8*
    malfunction of, 11–13
    survival and, 11
pain-relieving devices, 26
pain specialists, xvi, 33, 130, 186–87, 204, 211
pain tolerance, 9
Pamelor (nortriptyline), 45, 58, 76, 78, 136, 138, 154
pamindronate (Aridea), 97
pancreatic cancer, 200
panic attacks, 46, 47–48
paroxetine (Paxil), 46
partial facetectomy, 126
Patton, George, 158, 184

Paxil (paroxetine), 46
pelvic fracture, 130
pelvic inflammatory disease (PID), 176,
    177, 178–79
pelvic pain, 30, 173–84
    chronic, 174–75, 176–83
    recurrent, 175–76
    see also specific conditions
Percoset (oxycodone), 40, 54, 56–57,
    140, 192, 197
peroneal tendinitis, 162
Pert, Candice, 51
PET scan (isotope-based positron
    emission tomography), 15
phantom-limb pain, 141, 152–56
    prevention of, 155–56
    treatment for, 154–55
phenytoin (Dilantin), 47, 133, 139
physiatrists, 27, 211, 212
physical examination, 3–4, 13, 14, 15,
    16, 107
physical-fitness programs, 21
physical therapy, xvi, 4, 26–27, 31, 33,
    36, 38, 85, 89, 188
physicians, xv, xvi, 15, 16, 26
    fees of, 221
    selection of, 210–14
pillows, 20, 22
placebo effect, 145–46
plantar fasciitis, 162
Plaquenil (hydroxychloroquine), 94
pneumonia, 96
posterior parametritis, 176
postherpetic neuralgia, 147–49
posture, 17, 24
    changes of, 10, 19
    for driving, 20
premenstrual syndrome (PMS), 69,
    173, 175
prilocaine, 49
prostaglandins, 92–93
prostate, enlargement of, 46, 138
prostate cancer, 199
Prozac (fluoxetine), 46, 69
pruritus vulvae, 182
psychiatrists, 32–33, 76
psychologists, 32–33
psychosomatic medicine, xvi
psychotherapy, 28, 31–33, 76

radiation therapy, 134–35, 189–91,
    211–12
radiofrequency, 133–34, 144, 198,
    200

radiofrequency lesioning, 119–21, 124,
    200
radiological studies, v, 15, 186
raloxifene hydrochloride (Evista), 97
receptors, 4–5, 6, 12, 52
Reeve, Christopher, 166
reflex sympathetic dystrophy (RSD), 141
relaxation response, 27, 28, 29, 33, 38,
    71, 92
rest, ice, compression, and elevation
    (RICE), 160, 161, 171, 172
rheumatoid arthritis, 1, 31, 50, 91,
    94–95
rheumatologists, 97, 211
Rideau, Mariana, 122–23
rizatriptan (Maxalt), 68
rotator-cuff tendinitis, 162
running:
    long-distance, 21
    marathon, 21, 101

sacroiliac joint, 14, 109
    irritation of, 13
sacrum, 103
salmon calcitonin (Calcimar;
    Myacalcin), 97
sarcoma, 188–89
Schwarzenegger, Arnold, 40
sciatica, 2, 11, 35, 86, 90, 111–12,
    115, 116, 123–24, 168–69
sciatic nerve, irritation of, 13, 168–69
scoliosis, 106, 123, 126–27
second opinions, 14
selective serotonin receptor inhibitors
    (SSRIs), 46
sensitization, 11–13, 130
serotonin, 8, 45, 67
sertraline (Zoloft), 46
Seventh Congress for the International
    Society for the Study of Vulvar
    Disease, 181
sexual dysfunction, 46, 78, 136, 177,
    182–83
shingles, 45, 47, 146–49
shoulder:
    "frozen," 27, 188
    pain in, 13, 37
Simons, D. G., 86
sin, expiation of, xvi
sinusitis, 37, 38
skiing, 21, 92
skin, 4, 9
    laser energy to, 35
    supersensitivity of, 137

skin creams, 49–50
Skinner, B. F., 28
skydiving, 21
sleep, 22
    body positions for, 17, 20
    disturbances of, 24, 44, 45, 46, 67
    promotion of, 46
    time zone changes and, 24
sleepiness, 42, 56, 61, 136
Smith, Quentin, 130
smoking, 37
Snyder, Solomon, 51
social problems, 4, 31–32
social workers, 32
sodium channel blockers, 48
sodium hyaluronate (Hyalen), 93
spinal cord, 4, 5, 6, 8, *105*, 106, 109
    compression of, 37, *108*
    growth of, 12
    injuries of, 45, 151–52
    lesions of, 199
    pain impulses received in, 12–13, 41
    reflex mechanism of, 7
    tumors on, 44, 89, 100
spinal cord stimulation (SCS), 156
spinal disorders, v, 26
spinal fluid, *105*, 118
spinal fusions, 126–28
spinal slippage, 25, 128
spinal surgery, 2, 124–28
spine, 101–9, *102, 103, 105, 108*
    cervical, 101, *102, 103,* 104, *105,*
        108
    coccyx in, 101
    injuries of, 166
    lumbar, 101, *102, 103,* 104, *105,*
        109–11, *110, 111,* 112, *112*
    sacrum in, 101, *102, 103*
    thoracic, 101, *102, 103,* 104, *105,*
        109
    vertebrae of, 101–4, *102, 103*
spine pain, 4, 13, 14
spondylolysis, 167
sports injuries, 158–72
    emergency procedures for, 171
    key points about, 172
    overuse, 161–62
    prevention of, 21, 170–72
    sprains and strains as, 159–61
    treatment of, 21, 160, 161, 170–72
sports medicine, 159, 161
spray and stretch procedure, 87
SSRIs (selective serotonin receptor
    inhibitors), 46

staphylococcus bacteria, 178
stenosis, 128
steroids, 22, 44, 70, 188, 193
stoicism, xvi, 11, 40
stomach, 25
    irritation of, 2, 24, 43, 44
streptococcus bacteria, 178
stress, reduction of, 17
stress fractures, 163–64
stroke, 27, 37–38, 45, 138
    neuropathic pain of, 2, 151–52
    risk factors for, 25, 37
sub-acute pain, 2
substance P, 8, 12, 49–50
suicide, 42, 131
sumatriptan (Imitrex), 68, 70
support groups, 92
surgery, xv, 38
    back, 124–28
    decompressive, 37
    joint-replacement, 25
    pain following, 2, 10, 25, 30, 39,
        187–89
    pain-relieving, 18
    physical therapy following, 26–27
    repetition of, 25
    risks of, 116
sweating, 2
sympathectomy, 154–55
Synvisc, 93

Taxol, 192
Tegretol (carbamazepine), 47, 132–33,
    139, 154
temperature, 40
temporomandibular joint syndrome
    (TMJ), 2, 30, 45, 76–78
tendinitis, 161
tendons, 18, 160, 162
tennis elbow, 159, 160
tenosynovitis, 161–62
TENS, *see* transcutaneous electrical
    nerve stimulation
testicular cancer, 191
test-negative pain, 3–4, 14–15, 76
    conditions suggestive of, 14–15, 64,
        78, 131
    treatment for, 4
tests, xvi
    experimental, 15
    inadequacy of, 15
    minimally invasive, 14, 16
    see also specific tests
thalamus, 5, 6

therapeutic pillows, 20, 22
therapeutic touch, 36
thoracotomy, 187–88
throbbing, 9, 16, 41, 73
tic douloureux, 131–35
    treatment of, 132–35
tilted uterus, 177
tingling, 2, 30, 109
TMJ (temporomandibular joint
        syndrome), 2, 30, 45, 76–78
Tofranil (imipramine), 45
Tonocard (tocainide), 48
toothaches, 2, 14
total–body pain, 13
touch:
    excessive sensitivity to, 11, 130
    therapeutic, 36
tramadol (Ultram), 48, 140
transcendental meditation, 27
transcutaneous electrical nerve
        stimulation (TENS), 29–31, 33,
        35, 36, 87, 89, 116–17, 148, 154,
        156, 181, 189, 213
trauma, 27
    head, 78–84
    pain and, 2, 4, 11, 35, 70–73
travel, 22–25
    automobile, 2, 20, 23
    carrying baggage and, 22–24
    medications and, 24
    plane, 22–23
    time zone changes and, 24
Travell, Janet, 86
tricyclic antidepressants, 42, 45–46, 48,
        58, 69, 76, 136, 138–39, 143
trigeminal neuralgia, 131–35
    treatment of, 132–35
trigger-point injections, 35, 87
triptans, 68
    see also specific drugs
tumor necrosis factor, 95
tumors, 11, 14, 37, 44, 65
    bone, 3, 40
    brain, 44, 131
    fibroid, 179
    radiation-induced, 135
    spinal cord, 44, 89, 100
Tylenol (acetaminophen), xvi, 40, 42,
        57, 71, 93, 140, 170

ulcers, 43, 44
Ultram (tramadol), 48, 140
ultrasound stimulation, 87, 89, 117
urinary tract disorders, 177
urologists, 136, 173
uterine cancer, 97

vago-glossopharyngeal neuralgia,
        132–33
Valium-like drugs, 54, 78, 133, 148
valproic acid (Depakote), 47, 48, 69,
        133
vascular problems, 41
venlaxafine (Effexor), 46
vertebroplasty, 98–100, 201
Vicodin, 140
Vincristine, 192
Vioxx, 44
visceral pain, 2
vision loss, 25
vitamin D, 97
vomiting, 24, 51, 56, 67
vulvar pain syndrome, 181–82
vulvar vestibulitis, 181

walking, 24
    comfortable shoes for, 23
    as therapy, 26
water retention, 43, 44
weakness, 22, 25, 26, 37–38
weight:
    distribution of, 19–20, 22–24
    excess, 25, 44, 46, 92
    and lack of exercise, 25
    monitoring of, 19, 21, 25
    poor eating habits and, 25
Welbutrin (buproprion), 46
well-being, sense of, 4
whiplash injury, 4, 14, 74, 75
wincing, 2, 11
workplace injuries, 18

X rays, 15, 37, 73, 77, 79, 89, 96, 98,
        99, 114

zolmitriptan (Zomig), 68
Zoloft (sertraline), 46
Zostrix (capsaicin), 49–50, 139